AIDS:
Policies and Programs for the Workplace

AIDS:
Policies and Programs for the Workplace

Kathleen C. Brown, R.N., Ph.D.
Professor and Director of Occupational Health Nursing
NIOSH Deep South Center for
Occupational Safety and Health
University of Alabama at Birmingham

Joan G. Turner, R.N., Ph.D.
Professor and Director of Infection Control
Nurse Clinician Project
University of Alabama School of Nursing
University of Alabama at Birmingham

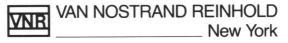
VAN NOSTRAND REINHOLD
New York

Printed in the United States of America

Van Nostrand Reinhold
115 Fifth Avenue
New York, New York 10003

Van Nostrand Reinhold International Company Limited
11 New Fetter Lane
London EC4P 4EE, England

Van Nostrand Reinhold
480 La Trobe Street
Melbourne, Victoria 3000, Australia

Macmillan of Canada
Division of Canada Publishing Corporation
164 Commander Boulevard
Agincourt, Ontario M1S 3C7, Canada

16 15 14 13 12 11 10 9 8 7 6 5 4 3 2 1

Library of Congress Cataloging in Publication Data

Brown, Kathleen C., 1946–
    AIDS, policies and programs for the workplace / Kathleen Brown
Joan G. Turner
        p. cm.
    Includes index.
    ISBN 0-442-23353-1
    1. AIDS (Disease)—Prevention.   2. Industrial hygiene.   3. Health
education.   4. Employee rights.   I. Turner, Joan G.   II. Title.
RA644.A25B76   1989
362.1'9697'92—dc19   89-5324

To Harry who gave us THE idea and shared the journey—K. B.

This one is especially for the 3647 Menagerie—J. T.

CONTENTS

viii   Contents

x   Contents

PREFACE

This book is about AIDS and workplace issues. Contagion, liability, health insurance, company policy, and screening are common issues for workers and employers alike. How do you get AIDS? Can I catch it at work? What will happen to my job and insurance if I am antibody positive? What company policy should we write? How do we manage an employee with AIDS? The Fortune 500 and Allstate *1988 Business Response to AIDS: A National Survey of U.S. Companies* reported that two-thirds of companies are currently concerned about AIDS and 84 percent will be concerned within the next five years. Yet, most companies are in dire need of guidance to help them develop company policy and educational programs on AIDS.

We have written this book to reduce the number of AIDS and workplace unknowns and to provide a compendium of AIDS information that will help companies and employees respond to the AIDS crisis rationally. Potential readers of this book include the working public, company managers, business owners, and occupational health professionals. No other comprehensive source of information has been published that covers occupational exposure to the HIV virus, worker protection, and workplace issues from a manager's perspective. We anticipate that workers concerned about occupational exposure to AIDS will read this book to learn about protection and what to expect from their employers. Company managers, human resource managers, and supervisors will use this book as a reference manual in planning a proactive corporate response to AIDS. For occupational health professionals, this book provides a current overview of facts on AIDS plus specifics regarding AIDS policies, education, screening, prevention, and care of the HIV-infected employee.

The book begins with current epidemiologic information and trends regarding AIDS contagion and prevention and a discussion of the financial impact of AIDS on business and society. It then goes on to a comprehensive description of formulating workplace AIDS policies, AIDS screening, and planning and conducting AIDS educational programs at the worksite. The legal implications of AIDS, workers' attitudes and fears regarding coworkers with AIDS, and management of the HIV-infected employee are presented in detail. A chapter on protecting workers from potential occupational exposure to AIDS is a unique feature of this book. In addition, the public relations and media perspective on AIDS is covered. Extensive material is presented to help the reader understand our nation's large-scale public health AIDS prevention and control efforts. Finally, a complete series of federal guidelines and workplace recommendations on AIDS is featured in this book.

ACKNOWLEDGMENTS

A major influence for us has been the inspiration and encouragement we have received from Bernadine Kuchinski at NIOSH, Vernon Rose at the University of Alabama at Birmingham, and our occupational health ERC counterparts at universities nationwide. Thanks to all of you.

Our gratitude is extended to Geraldine Williamson, editor of the *American Association of Occupational Health Nurses Journal*, for asking us to edit and contribute information on AIDS in the July 1988 special issue on AIDS. We are indebted to all the authors of those manuscripts reprinted in part in this book with permission of Slack Publishing Company and the *AAOHN Journal*; these include Wendy Booth, Hala Fawal, Dorothy Gauthier, Beverly Hansen, Rebecca Langner, Martha Long, Karen Newman, Joe Packa, Peggy Rivers, Ann Sirles, and Kenny Williamson.

We never forget that we would not be writing today if it were not for release time and administrative support. Jean Kelley, Associate Dean of our graduate programs, provided an intellectual climate that encourages writing activities. We are thankful for the opportunity to work with colleagues and students who reward us for our accomplishments in occupational health and infection control.

Thanks are also given to the American Red Cross, the *American Journal of Public Health*, the Centers for Disease Control, the *American Association of Occupational Health Nurses Journal*, the *Public Relations Journal*, and the Citizens Commission on AIDS for New York City and Northern New Jersey for permitting us to incorporate their materials in this book.

At Van Nostrand Reinhold, we want to single out and thank Bob Esposito for challenging us to write a timely occupational health book that will benefit workers, managers, and occupational health professionals.

A special note of thanks is due to Mike Carlson and Chuck Michelini for the expert chapters they contributed. Last, we want to acknowledge and thank family and friends who love and sustain us each and every day.

1.

FACTS ABOUT AIDS

From 1981, when the first cases were reported, to 1988, acquired immunodeficiency syndrome (AIDS) has been diagnosed in over 70,000 Americans. Although life expectancy is slowly increasing, 56 percent of all cases, or around 40,000 people, have died thus far, and the projected statistics for the next few years are grim.

By 1991, 270,000 total cases of AIDS are expected, and 179,000 persons in this country alone will have died. Further, in the year 1991 alone, 74,000 new cases of AIDS will be diagnosed, and at least 145,000 persons with AIDS are expected to be living and/or working in the United States. Currently, an estimated one to two million Americans are infected with the AIDS virus, and in the midst of ignorance, apathy and denial, that number increases incautiously and mercilessly.

Some level of AIDS has been reported in all major areas of the world. Although the United States has reported 70 percent of all cases worldwide, reporting from other areas of the world such as Africa is often incomplete and delayed. In fact, many people in places like Africa have no access to health-care facilities, and so they sicken, die, and are buried without treatment or diagnosis. Between 5 percent and 25 percent of women of childbearing age are known to be already infected in some urban parts of Central and East Africa. Societal reactions to AIDS in African countries have been similar to those in Europe and North America. Denial, panic, and stigmatization occur, and the United States is sometimes "blamed" for the AIDS epidemic, even though some evidence exists that the AIDS virus was present in Africa before it appeared in the United States. Because AIDS impacts most heavily on young and middle-aged adults, including members of the business and government elite, it brings with it a potential for worldwide economic and political destabilization where the virus is most common (Piot, Plummer & Mhalu, 1988).

To understand how these predictions can be made and what the ramifications are for society in general and the workplace in particular, this chapter explores the growing body of knowledge related to AIDS, the virus that precipitates the disease process, and the people it affects. Additionally, AIDS must be viewed within an evolutionary sense; that is, AIDS is not the only "new" infectious disease to affect humans, nor will it be the last. Examples of other infectious diseases recognized in recent years include genital herpes, Legionnaire's disease, toxic shock syndrome, and a new type of hepatitis that is almost uniformly fatal.

To begin to understand a phenomenon like AIDS, we have to appreciate the fact that germs or microbes are also living, evolving, and interacting with all other living things and physical forces that make up our universe. We have little trouble accepting the fact that most horticultural pests are now, in essence, immune to old pesticides like DDT, or that other small but visible pests like the killer bee or the fire ant have undergone changes in their physical structure and behavior to become even greater nuisances.

Why then do we have so much trouble understanding that microbes or microorganisms (literally meaning "living beings too small to be seen with the naked eye") also change? In fact, microorganisms are known to become resistant or "immune" to various antibiotics, and many microorganisms that formerly caused disease only in plants or animals now cause disease in humans. They have adapted or evolved to that point.

HUMAN IMMUNODEFICIENCY VIRUS

AIDS, and many AIDS-related conditions that will be subsequently explored, are initiated by infection with the human immunodeficiency virus (HIV). As its name reflects, HIV is a virus that affects a human's immune system, which is responsible for fighting off infection and/or making us "immune" to certain diseases. When the immune system is impaired, as it is when a person has any AIDS-related condition, the person loses an ability to repel invading substances like disease-causing microbes. So the first point is that people do not die of AIDS, they die because infection with HIV initially compromises their immune systems, and death results because the immune system may stop functioning to fight off infections. Failure of any bodily system is ultimately lethal, although some manifestations of system failure can be managed for a period of time by various medical interventions.

The human immunodeficiency virus is a member of a unique family of viruses called *retroviruses*. For the sake of simplicity, microorganisms are grouped into categories based on their chemical and/or organic properties, just as automobiles are classified into numerous categories according to size, weight, and design. A unique quality of the retrovirus is that one of its enzymes, reverse transcriptase, allows it to actually become a genetic part of the white blood cell during the infection process. Like all viruses, HIV is unable to reproduce or cause any damage until it enters a human cell.

Even though AIDS is believed to be a relatively new disease, scientists have known about the existence of retroviruses for more than 70 years. At first, retroviruses were of interest primarily to veterinarians because all known retroviruses caused disease in animals such as chickens and sheep. In fact, one retroviral disease that is familiar to most cat owners is feline leukemia, for which a preventive vaccine is now available. Cats do not transmit feline leukemia to humans any more than humans could transmit AIDS to cats, but both causative viruses are nevertheless classified as retroviruses.

In 1980, the first human retrovirus, one that caused a leukemia-like illness, was discovered. Since then, several other retroviruses that cause disease in humans have been discovered, but we will deal primarily with HIV because it is the virus that precipitates most AIDS-related illnesses in the United States.

AIDS-RELATED CONDITIONS

As mentioned previously, AIDS is not a disease. It is a syndrome that ranges all the way from early and silent infection to mild illnesses manifested by swollen lymph glands and weight loss to rare but lethal infections and cancer. When referring to the overall phenomenon of AIDS, ranging from infection to death, the use of the term AIDS-related conditions is appropriate. By definition, AIDS-related conditions or AIDS-related diseases refer to the entire spectrum of clinical and subclinical disease initiated by infection with HIV. For example, AIDS-related complex (ARC) and generalized lymphoadenopathy syndrome (GLS) were considered different disease manifestations produced by HIV infection. Since 1987, however, the Centers for Disease Control (CDC) changed the criteria for diagnosis, and now separate diagnoses are of interest to medical treatment teams. For our purposes, we will refer to AIDS-related conditions or AIDS-related diseases.

To begin with, the person infected with HIV may experience or manifest a variety of symptoms, or the individual may have no symptoms for several years. Most people infected with HIV probably do not know they are infected. In fact, HIV, like all infectious diseases, is associated with an incubation period, or the time interval beginning when the offending microbe actually enters the body and establishes itself, and the time when the disease can be detected or sensed in the form of signs and/ or symptoms. For example, when foods contaminated with some disease-causing microbe are eaten, usually no immediate reaction occurs to indicate that infection has taken place. When symptoms like abdominal cramping, diarrhea, nausea, and vomiting occur hours later, the incubation period has lapsed and the unfortunate person becomes aware that something is very wrong.

Yet, before we discuss incubation periods any further, we should make the point that exposure to HIV does not necessarily result in infection. Scientists learned in developing the germ theory that an organism (microbe) is *necessary but not sufficient* to cause disease; that is, although no one can contract any infectious disease unless exposed in the appropriate manner to the microbe that causes the disease, not everyone who is exposed becomes infected.

Why some exposures result in infection and others do not is not fully understood, but this lack of understanding is not unique to AIDS-like illnesses. For instance, not all sexual contacts of a prostitute who has a sexually transmitted disease like gonorrhea will also become infected. In fact, only about one in three contacts with diseases like gonorrhea or hepatitis actually result in infection. Even though male-to-female transmission is at least twice as efficient as female-to-male in a sexually transmitted disease, a male infected with gonorrhea, syphilis, herpes, or AIDS does not infect all sexual partners with whom he has contact (Rosenberg & Weiner, 1988). The AIDS virus has shown itself to be less capable of causing infection after exposure than most other known diseases. For example, Padian and associates (1987) found that 75 of 97 female sexual partners of HIV-infected men had not been infected by sexual contact.

A similar phenomenon has been observed in blood transfusion recipients in that only about half of the people who have received HIV-infected blood have subsequently become infected. The reasons are not clear but probably relate to the overall health status of the individual exposed to infection.

In general, a person's ability to repel potential infection when exposed to the causative microbe is probably related to the quality of the individual's health, the lack of immunosuppressive substances like alcohol, and even their genetic or inherited physical makeup. The importance of this discussion lies in the fact that the probability of any given person contracting any infectious disease like AIDS depends on: (1) coming in contact with the causative microbe in a fashion that allows infection and (2) the individual's resistance or susceptibility to infection.

Incubation Period

To return to the discussion on incubation periods, note that different diseases have characteristic but slightly different incubation periods. Although some diseases such as hepatitis and rabies may take months from exposure and infection until symptoms of disease develop, other diseases such as influenza have incubation periods of a few days. Finally, some diseases like food poisoning have an incubation period of only hours. Although talking about "incubation periods" in conjunction with chronic diseases like cancer or diabetes is generally inappropriate, these kinds of diseases may develop over many years or even a lifetime.

When speaking directly to diseases caused by HIV, referring to two different incubation periods is appropriate, simply because the infection can be detected long before the infected person has any reason to think something is physically wrong. So the first incubation period associated with AIDS is that period of time from initial infection until the time that infection can be detected by a combination of the ELISA and the Western blot blood tests. These tests are discussed at length in chapter 4.

At our current level of technology, the general agreement is that evidence of HIV infection can be detected by the ELISA and Western blot between 3 and 24 weeks after actual exposure and subsequent infection, but this time interval may extend to 12 months or more in some individuals. However, the period between initial infection and development of various AIDS-related conditions, including clinical AIDS, is long and variable.

The incubation period, or the time between infection and onset of symptoms, probably varies with the mode of transmission (the way in which a person becomes infected), the age, sex, and susceptibility of the person, and certainly the concentration of virus transmitted. Repeated exposure to HIV apparently greatly increases a person's chances of becoming infected. Additionally, some HIV-infected persons may be more efficient transmitters than others, and infectiousness may also vary in time over the course of the infection (Curran, Jaffee, Hardy, et al.,1988).

The incubation period is notably shorter in infants and women and is also shorter when the mode of transmission is intravenous, like a blood transfusion. Several studies have shown the incubation period in homosexual men who become infected through various types of sexual contact to be between 5 and 7 years, whereas infection from blood transfusion usually manifests itself in five years or less. In some adult sexually transmitted cases (either homosexual or heterosexual) the average incubation period may be as long as 15 years (Chavigny, Turner & Kibrick, 1988). At this point, whether everyone who is infected will ultimately develop disease is unknown, but current thinking indicates that most HIV-infected people will ultimately experience some AIDS-related condition.

Symptoms

The earliest symptom—experienced by some persons within weeks of infection with HIV—is a flulike syndrome that may be accompanied by a generalized rash. When it occurs—and it does not always occur nor is it noticed in many cases—it lasts only a few days as with any flulike syndrome, and the person then returns to the usual state of health. Most infected individuals do not experience AIDS-related symptoms for years. Regardless of symptoms, however, once infection with HIV occurs, the affected person also becomes infectious; that is, even with no symptoms, the infected person is believed to be capable of infecting others through sexual or blood contact for life. Either medicines or vaccines may be developed at some point in the future that would act to make the person noninfectious to others, but for now that technology does not exist and has not been scientifically demonstrated.

Symptoms associated with the onset of AIDS-related conditions include:

- Enlarged lymph nodes in the neck, under the arm, or in the groin that persist for a long period of time
- Persistent fever or fevers developing in the afternoon or evening
- Involuntary loss of weight
- Fatigue
- Diarrhea that cannot be explained and does not respond to usual over-the-counter medications
- Purplish, irregularly shaped spots on the skin or in the mouth
- A white, cheesy coating on the tongue or in the mouth
- Night sweats
- Forgetfulness or change in personality

Whenever one or more of these symptoms is experienced, the individual should consult a health-care provider for at least two reasons. First, all the symptoms indicate that the individual's health status is compromised, and the problem may or may not be precipitated by HIV infection. If the reason for any of the above symptoms is not related to HIV infection, this knowledge could come as a tremendous relief for the individual. Second, anyone who is HIV infected needs to know it in order to take measures to avoid infecting others through sex, childbirth, or blood or organ donation. Also, the HIV-infected person needs to do anything in his or her power to enhance overall personal health, including adequate rest, proper nutrition, learning stress management, and, at all costs, avoiding reinfection. One therapeutic advantage to knowing whether or not one is infected is the fact that newly available drugs are thought to slow the action of the virus. One of these "antiviral" drugs, azidothymidine (commonly called AZT), has been approved by the federal Food and Drug Administration, and some clinical researchers believe best effects can be obtained from this drug when it is started fairly early in the course of infection. Although not all HIV-infected people can tolerate AZT (just as some people cannot take penicillin or aspirin), those who tolerate the drug may gain a variety of benefits such as fewer infections with longer relatively "healthy periods." AZT and other antiviral drugs may also decrease an infected person's ability to transmit HIV (Volberding, 1988).

Stages of Health Deterioration

Very little about the course of HIV infection is strictly predictable. As the preceding discussion pointed out, the incubation period is long and variable. Moreover, both initial occurrences of illnesses and the overall life expectancy of people with AIDS-related conditions will likely be altered by new drugs and treatment regimens. The following scenario was designed to show the relative chronological order of symptoms and illnesses experienced by people with AIDS to help the employer understand the physical and some emotional anomalies experienced by people with the disease.

The first phase spans the incubation period, or that time from initial infection to the onset of symptoms. The symptoms are the same as those recounted in the previous section and include night sweats, loss of weight, increasing fatigue, and fevers. Different people can tolerate such symptoms for varying periods of time. Additionally, if the health-care provider does not specifically test for evidence of HIV infection or does not take a very careful and sensitive health and sexual history, the diagnosis can be missed, and people may be told that they apparently have had some viral syndrome that will go away in time.

During this phase of early and vague symptomatology, the individual may react in any number of ways, depending upon whether he suspects exposure to HIV has occurred or not. Typically, the individual demonstrates some absenteeism from work. The individual also has a lessened ability to participate in social activities and feels a lot of confusion and fear regarding the cause of the symptoms.

Occupational health professionals who recognize these symptoms should be as supportive as possible while referring the employee to definitive diagnosis and treatment facilities. If the worker wishes to see a private physician, the referring appointment should be made in the presence of the employee, who can then commit to keeping the appointment.

As we point out again and again in this book, conducting ELISA and Western blot testing at the worksite is probably not advisable. If the worker wishes to be tested for evidence of HIV infection, this testing should be conducted at a site where complete pre- and post-test counseling is available, and confidentiality should be guaranteed. As discussed in chapter 4, free or low-fee confidential testing is available at most county health departments across the country. The individual who tests positive is told in person and seen on site by a qualified physician or referred to one of the individual's choice.

For the worker who tests positive for infection with HIV, one of the first and most difficult decisions is with whom to share the information. If the employee chooses to share this information with the employer, the employer must know that his or her first responsibility is maintaining the confidentiality of that disclosure (see chapter 6 for more detailed discussion of employer rights and responsibilities). At this point, the enlightened and humane employer assures the employee of confidentiality, and, if both parties seem ready, future provisions relative to the work setting could be discussed.

CHARACTERISTICS AND TRENDS ASSOCIATED WITH AIDS

HIV infection is transmitted by three routes: (1) sexual contact, (2) blood contact, and (3) mother to child during the
pregnancy or birthing period. Virtually any sexual act with
exchange of body fluids such as semen and/or vaginal secretions, whether homosexual or heterosexual, can result in
infection *if either partner is infected with HIV.*

Since May 1985, the blood industry has been required to test
each donated unit for evidence of HIV infection. When evidence of infection is found, the blood is discarded and the
donor is notified. Because of this testing for evidence of AIDS
and other diseases like hepatitis B, the American blood supply
is safer than ever before in history. Yet, the screening test
currently being used to detect HIV infectivity is not perfect (see
discussion in chapter 4), and, consequently, during an approximately three-week window or interval in the incubation period
no evidence of HIV may be detected. A great deal of research
is currently being directed at improving screening tests for HIV
infection. In addition, blood banks are conducting a conscien-
tious program of "self-deferral," in which potential donors are
urged to mark their data cards if they feel they may even be at
risk for HIV infection. The result, according to the American
Red Cross, is that less than one unit of blood in every 100,000
available for emergency transmission may conceivably be contaminated with HIV.

In the interest of perspective, to date, transfusion of whole
blood or blood components has resulted in fewer than 2,000
documented cases of AIDS, or about 3 percent of all cases
diagnosed. In addition, about 10,000 to 15,000 severe hemophiliacs in this country must receive clotting factor made from
thousands of units of plasma (the liquid portion of whole
blood). Although many hemophiliacs had been infected prior
to the blood screening that began in 1985, to date fewer than
700 cases of AIDS have been reported in this group.

By August 1988, nearly 1,100 cases of pediatric AIDS had
been reported in the United States. By definition, pediatric

AIDS includes those cases diagnosed in children under 13 years of age. Although children have been infected by receiving HIV-contaminated blood transfusions, and also through taking the blood-clotting medication needed by hemophiliacs, the vast majority of persons with pediatric AIDS were infected by their mothers.

Pregnancy should be deferred indefinitely in individuals known to be HIV infected. However, when HIV-infected women do become pregnant, their offspring have a fifty-fifty chance of developing full-blown AIDS shortly after birth. Even if the mother is not infected when she conceives, if she becomes infected during the course of the pregnancy, the child still has a 50 percent chance of developing AIDS. At this point, why babies born to infected mothers do or do not become infected and subsequently develop the disease is not understood.

Race

From a racial perspective, AIDS is a disease that affects minorities disproportionately—black and Hispanic adults and children have 3 to 12 times more cases of diagnosed AIDS than do whites in this country. Although blacks account for only 18 percent of the total U.S. population, 25 percent of all adult cases of AIDS and 56 percent of all pediatric AIDS cases have occurred in blacks. Hispanics, who are only 6.5 percent of the U.S. population, have accounted for 13 percent of the adult and 20 percent of all pediatric cases. In fact, the risk for blacks and Hispanics who live in the northeastern part of the country are 2 to 10 times greater than the risk for those who live in other areas because of the high concentration of intravenous (IV) drug abuse–related cases (Curran et al., 1988).

Age

The great majority of Americans who die from AIDS or AIDS-related conditions are in the 20- to 44-year-old age group (over

90 percent), and half are in the third decade of life. The median age of homosexual men with AIDS is 34; drug abusers tend to be younger, and blood-transfusion recipients older (Allen, 1984).

One measure of the premature mortality associated with AIDS is years of potential life lost (YPLL) before age 65. Most causes of YPLL decrease or increase only slightly over many decades, but AIDS increased from the thirteenth leading cause of YPLL in 1984 to the eighth leading cause in 1986. In 1988, AIDS ranked as the sixth leading cause of YPLL. More than 90 percent of AIDS-related premature mortality occurs in men because 90 percent of all cases of AIDS have been diagnosed in men (Curran et al., 1988).

Geographic Location

In addition to racial minorities being at greater risk of HIV infection in the northeastern United States, whites are also at greater risk in this part of the country. New York City alone has reported more than 15,000 cases of AIDS to CDC. On any given day, 1,200 people are hospitalized in New York City for AIDS-related diseases. A study late in 1987 demonstrated that about 1 in 60 babies born in city hospitals showed evidence of HIV infection in either the child or the mother. One of its neighboring cities, Jersey City, has reported almost 1,000 pediatric and adult cases, and Newark, New Jersey, has reported nearly 2,000 cases. To date, AIDS cases have been concentrated in large cities that also have large populations of homosexual and bisexual men and IV drug addicts. However, the prediction early in 1988 from CDC was that larger numbers of future AIDS cases would appear in what are currently areas of low incidence.

HIV-Infection Through Sexual Contact

Although roughly 80 percent of all cases of AIDS have occurred in either homosexual or bisexual men or IV drug users, as of July 1988, 2,859 persons (1,234 men, 1,625 women) in the United States had ostensibly contracted AIDS through heterosexual contact (Centers for Disease Control, 1988). Despite indicators that new infections with HIV among gay and bisexual men are sharply declining, the number of heterosexually acquired cases is slowly but steadily increasing to about 7 percent of all cases of AIDS reported to CDC in 1988.

The two primary mechanisms by which HIV is spread heterosexually is through contact with bisexuals and IV drug users. For example, a significant portion of prostitutes are believed either to be themselves IV drug users or to have regular sexual partners who use drugs. As prostitutes become infected, they become capable of transmitting infection to others.

The other group that promotes spread of HIV infection to the heterosexual population is bisexual men, who by definition have sexual contact with both men and women. Although their numbers are factually unknown, CDC estimates between 2.5 and 7.5 million bisexual men in the United States (Centers for Disease Control, 1987). Further, some argue that bisexual men could be at greater risk of becoming HIV infected than those who are exclusively homosexual simply because the bisexual male may enter the gay community for the express purpose of finding a readily available sexual contact. That "readily available" sexual contact may be a male prostitute or sexually a very promiscuous individual. Once infected, the bisexual is then capable of infecting subsequent male and female sexual partners.

Numerous studies have been conducted in the United States on high-risk groups such as homosexual and bisexual men, IV drug users, and prostitutes. Using the blood test explained in chapter 4, convenience samples have yielded alarming levels of infectivity as indicated by seropositivity of their blood. For example, more than 50 studies since 1984 have shown that 10 percent to 70 percent (with most between 20 percent and 50 percent) of homosexual and bisexual men were already infected. The infection rate among IV drug users was much more variable, ranging from none to 70 percent, with rates generally higher in the major East Coast cities (Curran et al., 1988). Rates of infectivity among prostitutes vary from none to 45 percent with the highest rates occurring in large inner cities where IV drug use is common (Centers for Disease Control, 1987). Other more recent reports say that infectivity among prostitutes ranges between zero and 65 percent (Rosenberg & Weiner, 1988).

HIV INFECTIVITY AMONG THE U.S. POPULATION AT LARGE

One way we can get a feel for the level of HIV infectivity among the overall population of the United States is to look at data generated by testing for the AIDS virus in all recruits to military and Peace Corps service. From over 1 million such applicants, we have learned that males are infected two or three times more often than females. Black applicants are three to seven times more likely to be infected, as are those recruits who come from areas with a greater number of AIDS cases, such as the Northeast. For example, one of 50 recruits (2 percent) from New York City's borough of Manhattan were infected (Griggs, 1986). However, recruits who show evidence of HIV infectivity are still relatively rare in some parts of the country. Overall, fewer than one person in 1,000 is expected to be HIV infected, but seroprevalence studies now in progress will be able to verify or negate that rate.

WHO IS AT RISK OF HIV INFECTION?

The great majority of Americans do not "shoot" IV drugs nor engage in homosexual activity, but they are sexually active. The only safe sex from an infectious disease standpoint is that which takes place in a long-term, mutually monogamous relationship in which neither of the partners is HIV infected. Outside a mutually monogamous relationship, the only sure way to avoid HIV infection is to be sexually abstinent. The remainder of this discussion is addressed to those sexually active people who occasionally or regularly engage in sexual liaisons outside the long-term, mutually monogamous relationship.

The first truism relative to risk for HIV infection in the sexually active, nonmutually monogamous American is that risk increases as the number of partners increases, especially if partners are not chosen very carefully. Two AIDS researchers, Hearst and Hulley (1988), recently reported that sexually active adults should, above all else, be taught to choose their sexual partners from people they know to be at very low risk of carrying HIV infection. Persons at high risk for HIV infection include: (1) anyone who within the past ten years has engaged in homosexual activity or IV drug use, (2) people who have a history of multiple blood transfusions, (3) sexually promiscuous persons, (4) hemophiliacs, and (5) anyone who has had a sexual partner in any of the first four groups.

One of the obvious problems with advising people to avoid high-risk sexual partners is that some people might be unaware that a past sexual partner was, for example, bisexual. Some people might purposefully choose to withhold such things in their past. When in doubt about a sexual partner, using a condom with spermicidal jelly and avoiding anal intercourse may be helpful (Hearst & Hulley, 1988).

SUMMARY

The purpose of this introductory chapter was to acquaint the reader with the general body of knowledge relative to AIDS and AIDS-related conditions. Basic mechanisms of transmission were elaborated, as were the characteristics of people that place them at high risk of infection.

REFERENCES

Allen, J. R. (1984) Epidemiology: United States. In P. Ebbe-
    sen, R. J. Biggar & M. Melbye, eds., *AIDS: A Basic
    Guide for Clinicians*, pp. 15–28. Philadelphia: W. B.
    Saunders.
Centers for Disease Control (1988) *AIDS Weekly Surveillance
    Report—United States.* July 25, Atlanta.
Centers for Disease Control (1987) Human immunodefi-
    ciency virus infection in the U.S.: A review of current
    knowledge. *Morbidity and Mortality Weekly Report*
    36(49):1–48.
Chavigny, K. H., L. S. Turner & A. K. Kibrick (1988) Epidemi-
    ology and health policy imperatives for AIDS. *New
    England Journal of Health Policy,* (special issue on
    AIDS), 4(1):59–79.
Curran, J. W., H. W. Jaffee, A. M. Hardy, et al. (1988) Epi-
    demiology HIV infection and AIDS in the United
    States. *Science,* 239:610–616.
Griggs, J., ed. (1986) *AIDS: Public Policy Dimensions.* New
    York: United Hospital Fund of New York.
Hearst, N. & S. B. Hulley (1988) Preventing heterosexual
    spread of AIDS: Are we giving our patients the best
    advice? *Journal of the American Medical Association*
    259 (16):2428–2432.
Padian, N., L. Marquis & D. P. Frances (1987) Male-to-
    female transmission of human immunodeficiency
    virus. *Journal of the American Medical Association*
    258:788–790.
Piot, P., F. A. Plummer & F. S. Mhalu (1988) AIDS: An inter-
    national perspective. *Science* 239 (1):573–579.
Rosenberg, M. J., & J. M. Weiner (1988) Prostitutes and
    AIDS: A health department priority. *American Journal
    of Public Health* 78(4):418–423.
Volberding, P. (1988) *HIV Disease Management: Issues and
    Answers* New York: World Health Communications,
    Inc.

2.
FINANCIAL IMPLICATIONS FOR BUSINESS AND SOCIETY

Anything that affects the health and well-being of a society also impacts on the production of goods and services. Therefore, the economic effect of AIDS, like the number of diagnosed cases, is just beginning to manifest itself. On the positive side, AIDS has acted as a stimulus for some industries like latex manufacturers, pharmaceutical development and research companies, and all manner of communication and/or mass media productions. Additionally, although no cure is yet available, significant technologic and scientific advances have been made as a result of efforts to understand (and hopefully some-day to control) the human immunodeficiency virus (HIV) and its malevolent family of human retroviruses. Yet, debts incurred while acting to prevent, control, and treat persons with AIDS (PWAs) mount every time another individual becomes infected.

The purpose of this chapter is to discuss the financial impact that AIDS-related diseases have had on business, private health and life insurance underwriters, the health-care delivery system, and the public sector. Because employment settings, large or small, are part of the greater governmental and private communities, federal, state, and local expenditures related to AIDS are discussed. Through this discussion the employer can gain an understanding of how health care for PWAs has and can be financed and how each workplace can act to reduce associated costs.

WHAT ARE THE HEALTH-CARE COSTS?

At least two reasons explain the difficulty of coming up with an accurate statement of cost associated with any phenomenon as wide-ranging and complex as AIDS-related diseases. First of all, to make accurate predictions, we need to know how many people will need treatment in a given time period. This criterion, in and of itself, is difficult because AIDS is a syndrome whereby an affected person may require no hospitalization one year but may need three or more admissions the next. The life span of people with HIV infection and related disorders is also highly variable. We are well aware that most people will not develop symptoms for five or more years after infection, but for every year beyond the first five after infection, more and more will succumb to the disease by manifesting symptoms of one kind of another. If we diagnose and treat promptly, less hospitalization is needed. If prompt diagnosis and treatment does not occur, life span could be significantly shortened.

So not only does the clinical picture of AIDS-related disease vary greatly, but also we are unsure how many Americans are infected and if and when they will become ill and require health care. The CDC's estimate is that between 1.2 and 1.8 million people are HIV infected in this country alone. Other estimates are higher. For example, researchers in Colorado have found that persons who are HIV infected outnumber

AIDS-diagnosed cases between 30 to one and 50 to one (Judson & Vernon, 1988). At our present rate of roughly 70,000 diagnosed cases, we would have between 2.1 million and 3.5 million Americans currently HIV infected.

The two estimates of infectivity among Americans is given not to alarm, nor to endorse the higher estimate, but to show the potential error involved when dealing with unknowns. In all fairness, the CDC estimates of the number infected are based on a sound mathematical model; additionally, their projections of the numbers of new AIDS cases have been exceedingly on target.

The other reason for the difficulty in projecting future health-care costs or even in comparing health-care costs between different patients, treatment care facilities, or even regions of the country is that so many uncontrollable variables enter to bias the resulting picture. First of all, as stands to reason and has been validated by research on a variety of diseases, outpatient management of virtually any health problem costs much less than inpatient treatment or hospitalization. That fact will be revalidated by the following discussion.

Another apparent truism is that hospital care is more costly in some regions of the country for treatment of AIDS-related conditions. For example, as we shall see, the lowest cost of hospitalization for PWAs is reported in San Francisco and the highest in the northeastern United States. We cannot automatically assume that hospital facilities and medical practitioners are more efficient or cost conscious in San Francisco because too many other factors might account for the differences. Suffice it to say that a study finding that has been reported more than once is that *experienced* medical teams—that is, health-care professionals who have more experience dealing with the uniquenesses of AIDS-related conditions—tend to deliver more cost-effective care.

Another factor that contributes to the cost-effectiveness of health-care delivery for PWAs is that the system in question works in close conjunction with community-based volunteer groups. These volunteers, when appropriately trained and managed, can perform small tasks that may make the difference in wellness or illness to a PWA. When the PWA is feeling too ill to obtain proper nutrition, a visiting volunteer can prepare a small meal and urge the individual to eat. For the PWA, maintaining adequate nutritional intake can mean the difference between living and dying. Perhaps the PWA is homebound and feeling too ill to travel to the drugstore to get a prescription renewed. In this case, the volunteer can either transport the client or run the errand, and certainly taking prescribed medication on time is one measure that prevents unnecessary hospitalization. The point is that the needs of PWAs are too diverse to be met by health-care professionals alone. Their efforts are greatly enhanced by the community volunteer approach. The salary cost of a community volunteer is much less than the cost of an hourly skilled or semiskilled employee.

Finally, another identifiable impact on the health-care cost for any illness is the introduction of newer technology and/or treatment regimens like medications. For example, if one compared the cost of health-care for patients in kidney failure who consent to renal dialysis to those who refuse dialysis, the cost would be higher for patients who chose the newer technological management. For one thing, patients on dialysis could live until they died of some other ailment, and those refusing the treatment would die in a very short time of kidney failure. The same is true of cancer patients, diabetics, and even organ transplant recipients. The cost is higher among those who avail themselves of technological breakthroughs.

Partially because AIDS-related diseases constitute a whole new realm of total body pathology, we can expect clients who choose to access newer treatments possibly to live longer and probably to cost the system—some system—more money than if the decision were made to go quietly off and die as soon as possible. If you have cared for a person with AIDS-related conditions, your beliefs about an individual's right to potentially effective (if expensive) treatments may be very favorable in this regard.

Many health-care institutions, especially acute-care hospitals, have found themselves in a precarious position during this escalating epidemic. One nationwide study of health-care costs found that the total annual costs for hospitalization of any given PWA was $20,320, of which only $15,424 was recovered by the treating institution (Abridge, 1988). Furthermore, on a national scale, CDC estimated that the 18,720 living Americans with AIDS required more than $380 million in hospital care in 1985, but $91.8 million of that amount was unrecoverable. This kind of deficit financing points to the wisdom of developing alternative, community-based treatment facilities for people with AIDS in an attempt to minimize unnecessary hospitalizations. But at the same time realistic payment strategies must be developed to reimburse professional services that emanate from these agencies. Without fair provision for payment from health insurance underwriters and medicaid, in light of the fact that a great proportion of PWAs are medically indigent, these community-based agencies would find that they were not recovering enough payment to remain operational.

Treatment with drugs like AZT is a mixed blessing, both from a clinical standpoint and from a cost perspective. Although AZT and other drugs may reduce the number of bouts with deadly pneumonias, AZT could backfire and result in more lifetime hospitalizations simply because these AIDS clients live longer (Landers & Seage, 1988). In addition, once individuals start on AZT, a two-year course of the drug is recommended if the dosage is tolerated. Because treated clients are healthier longer, however, they may also be able to work longer so that medical and social indigence is delayed or avoided.

COSTS ASSOCIATED WITH HOSPITALIZATION
VERSUS COMMUNITY-BASED MANAGEMENT

Studies conducted in Maryland, Massachusetts, New York, New Mexico, Alabama, Minnesota, Florida, Virginia, and California indicate that hospitalization over the lifetime of an AIDS-related disease patient costs $20,000 to $60,000 per patient. In Massachusetts, for example, an average hospital stay for a PWA was found to last 21 days and cost $14,189, which would interpret into an annual cost of $46,505. Another study of hospital charges done in Washington State reported a yearly average of $32,081 for care of PWAs (Lafferty et al., 1988).

We have already noted that caring for people with more advanced disease would be relatively more costly. To validate that notion, Seage and associates (1988) found that treatment for PWAs with mild symptoms such as swollen lymph glands and treatable diarrhea, without drugs like AZT cost as little as $489 per year, including professional fees and all ancillary use of the outpatient clinic.

A study done in San Francisco compared costs between hospital care and home care with appropriate support services including the aforementioned community-based organization. The authors reaffirmed the fact that when adequate services are available outside the hospital, the number of hospital days can be dramatically reduced, as can the accompanying financial outlay. Additionally, patient satisfaction was greater when managed with home health services. The estimate for acute inpatient management was between $500 and $800 per day, depending on treatments required. The comparable daily cost to care for a PWA in a extended-care facility such as a nursing home was $300 per day. The total cost of home support and nursing services from diagnosis to death was estimated at less than $5,000 per patient (Landers & Seage, 1988).

Direct Costs of AIDS

Direct costs attributable to AIDS include the personal medical costs previously discussed as well as nonpersonal costs such as research efforts, testing of blood and blood products for HIV, health education, and other support services such as those found within the community volunteer groups. We have seen that the cost of personal care is partially a function of where the disease is managed and certainly how the disease manifests itself and how many severe complications can be avoided through careful outpatient monitoring. We have also seen that high-quality, outpatient, community-based management is far more cost-effective than hospitalization for most conditions. So even though lifetime personal medical costs probably range somewhere between $20,000 and $60,000 per patient, the total cost in 1986 alone was $1.1 billion. That cost will increase to $8.5 billion in 1991 for personal health-care costs (Scitovsky & Rice, 1988).

The other part of direct costs attributable to AIDS consists of nonpersonal costs like research, blood testing, health education, and support services. These services carried a designated price tag in 1986 of $542 million and will rise in 1991 to $2.3 billion (Scitovsky & Rice, 1988). As an illustration of how costs associated with testing for evidence of the HIV virus account for millions of dollars, the total cost incurred by blood banks in 1986 for testing about 10 million blood donors was over $36 million (Eisenstaedt & Getzen, 1988).

Estimates of Indirect Costs

Estimates of indirect costs involve placing a monetary value on people's lost output because of a reduction or cessation in productivity caused by morbidity and mortality. Accordingly, morbidity costs are wages lost by people who are too sick to work or even to perform their usual housekeeping services. Mortality costs include the present value of future earnings lost by people who die prematurely. Morbidity costs in 1986 dollars for PWAs were $421 million in 1986 and will be $2.3 billion in 1991. The mortality cost attributable to AIDS in 1986 was about $5 billion, and for 1991 the mortality costs will rise to an estimated $30 billion.

PRIVATE INSURERS AND AIDS

Personal health-care costs associated with AIDS have elicited strong but variable responses from the private insurance sector and fairly open confrontation between the private versus the public sector insurers simply because (1) insurers wish to decrease their exposure to high costs, (2) companies do not want their premiums to rise, and (3) government health-care budgets need to remain responsive to a wide variety of political interests. Additionally, health maintenance organizations (HMOs) are concerned that PWAs or HIV-infected individuals will force their annual premiums up to the point where the facility may not be competitive with other forms of insurance that may offer more care-delivery options. A growing number of firms no longer offer common policies and are instead self-insuring. In fact, 85 percent of firms with over 40,000 employees and 70 percent of firms with 20,000 to 30,000 employees are now self-insured (Landers & Seage, 1988). The prospect of what PWAs will cost them is of great concern.

Many ethical, social, and economic phenomena have impacted heavily on the life and health insurance industry since the early 1980s, when soaring prime rates and double-digit investment returns led insurance companies with high capital pools into the equity, investment, and other risky markets. Even though expenditures on AIDS-related diseases have been relatively low to date compared with economic costs associated with other diseases, the fear (and the reality) is that costs associated with AIDS will be as high or higher than for previously known diseases.

Scitovsky and Rice (1988), two oft-cited medical economists, recently reported that the $7 billion for all indirect costs of AIDS in the United States in 1986 accounted for only 2.1 percent of all estimated total indirect costs of all illnesses. By 1991, however, AIDS-related indirect costs will be close to 12 percent of the total expenditure on illness, and the personal medical costs of AIDS in 1991 will be $8.5 billion, representing 1.4 percent of all personal health-care expenditures in

1991. The proportion of cost generated by AIDS would be reassuring if it were not growing at such a rate.

The cost of treating and dealing with AIDS is compounded by the fact that 50 million Americans currently have inadequate health-care coverage, and 30 million people under age 60 have none at all (McLaughlin, 1988). In general, workers in smaller and nonunionized firms are less likely to have employment-related coverage, but their household income may still be too high to qualify for programs like medicaid, which is intended to serve the indigent (Landers & Seage, 1988).

According to Lipson (1988), "The biggest problem in the AIDS crisis—for the insurance industry—is viability in the face of a swelling claims experience. The biggest problem for consumers, however, is protecting themselves from the insurance industry as it decides how it is going to cope with the crisis" (p. 286). Others in the insurance industry say that AIDS may become synonymous with bankruptcy. These spokespeople cite an average lifetime medical cost of $97,000 per patient (which is more than twice the highest range provided by economists), and the fact that the industry paid out $292 million in 1986 in AIDS-related death benefits alone.

In an effort to reduce the risks of underwriting life and health policies on what they consider "high-risk people," the private sector insurance industry has engaged in a variety of actions including refusing to underwrite individuals based on their sexual orientation and testing applicants for evidence of HIV infection. In fact, some insurers have terminated coverage upon learning that a given individual was tested but found negative for evidence of HIV infection. Insurers reasoned that the persons who seek testing are those persons who believe they are at high risk for the disease.

Such actions taken by insurance companies are essentially legal in many states. In fact, 43 states currently have no regulations prohibiting insurance underwriters from conducting HIV testing as a condition for eligibility for individual health insurance policies, but 22 states and the District of Columbia have written laws that forbid the inclusion of questions designed to

Table 2-1   STATE-IMPOSED HEALTH INSURANCE REGULATIONS PERTAINING TO HIV TESTING AND AIDS

State	Total Number AIDS Cases[a]	Forbid Questions Re: Prior Testing	Forbid Testing by Companies	Forbid Sexual Discrimination Based on Sexual Orientation	Forbid Exclusion of AIDS	Forbid Questioning of Group Applicants
New York[b]	10289	Yes	Yes	No	Yes	Yes
California[b]	7478	Yes	Yes	Yes	Yes	Yes
Florida[b]	2197	No	No	No	Yes	Yes
Texas[b]	2143	No	Yes	Yes	No	No
New Jersey[b]	1966	Yes	Yes	Yes	No	Yes
Illinois[b]	837	No	No	Yes	No	No
Pennsylvania[b]	752	No	No	Yes	Yes	No
Georgia[b]	688	No	No	Yes	Yes	Yes
Massachusetts[b]	680	Yes	Yes	Yes	No	Yes
D.C.[b]	624	Yes	Yes	Yes	Yes	
Maryland[b]	526	No	No	Yes	Yes	
Washington	410	No	No	No	No	
Louisiana	405	No	No	No	No	
Connecticut	395	Yes	No	No	No	
Virginia	388	No	No	No	No	
Colorado[b]	345	No	No	Yes	No	
Ohio[b]	302	No	No	No	No	
Michigan	293	Yes	Yes	Yes	Yes	
Missouri	213	No	No	No	Yes	
North Carolina	203	No	No	No	No	
Minnesota	178	Yes	No	Yes	Yes	
Arizona	174	Yes	Yes	Yes	Yes	
Indiana[b]	146	No	No	No	Yes	
Oregon	127	No	No	Yes	Yes	
Hawaii[b]	117	No	No	No	No	
South Carolina	117	No	No	No	No	
Wisconsin[b]	103	No	No	Yes	No	
Tennessee	101	No	No	Yes	Yes	

Table 2-1 (Continued)

State	Total Number AIDS Cases[a]	Forbid Questions Re: Prior Testing	Forbid Testing by Companies	Forbid Sexual Discrimination Based on Sexual Orientation	Forbid Exclusion of AIDS	Forbid Questioning of Group Applicants
Oklahoma	99	No	No	No	No	
Nevada	82	Yes	No	Yes	No	
Kentucky	77	No	No	No	No	
Alabama[b]	75	No	No	No	No	
Kansas	68	No	No	Yes	Yes	
Rhode Island	66	No	No	No	No	
Utah	59	No	No	No	No	
New Mexico	55	No	No	No	No	
Arkansas[b]	52	No	No	No	No	
Delaware	49	Yes	Yes	Yes	Yes	
Mississippi	45	No	No	No	No	
Iowa[b]	41	No	No	Yes	No	
Maine	40	Yes	No	No	No	
New Hampshire	27	No	No	No	No	
Alaska	25	No	No	No	No	
Nebraska	25	No	No	No	No	
West Virginia	22	No	No	No	No	
Vermont	11	No	No	No	No	
Idaho	8	No	No	No	No	
Montana	7	No	No	Yes	No	
Wyoming	7	No	No	No	No	
North Dakota[b]	4	No	No	Yes	No	
South Dakota	4	Yes	No	Yes	Yes	

From "Health Insurance and AIDS: The Status of State Regulatory Activity" by R.R. Faden and N.E. Kass, 1988, American Journal of Public Health, 78, p. 438. Reprinted by permission of the American Journal of Public Health.

[a] Cumulative total since June 1981 as reported to the CDC as of March 30, 1987.
[b] States contacted by the authors. All others contacted by the National Gay Rights Advocates.

identify the sexual orientation of applicants for health insurance. (See Table 2-1) Seventeen other states forbid health insurance companies from excluding AIDS as a covered medical condition after the policy is in force (Faden & Kass, 1988).

In effect, legislation affecting private insuring of PWAs and people at high risk for the disease varies widely, and thus far no federal laws have been enacted for the sake of standardization. Clearly, both the insurance industry and employers have legitimate business interests in protecting themselves from what they see as significant financial loss. Yet, the fact remains that if the private sector is permitted to eliminate or reduce AIDS-related costs from their share of the market, the implications for the public sector and the health-care industry may be staggering (Faden & Kass, 1988). One has only to be reminded that we are the only country in the industrialized world that does not have some form of national health insurance to contemplate the alternatives.

REDUCING COSTS

HIV infection is associated with an incubation period of five or more years from initial infection to onset of symptoms, and no vaccine introduced to prevent initial infection is likely to act to reverse the disease process. Treatments, mostly in the form of drugs, may act to lengthen life or even render the HIV-infected individual uninfectious, but as with our discussion of AZT, these drugs are likely to be expensive and may result in more long-term costs for medical care by extending life. The point is that the people who will be our AIDS cases in 1991 and 1992 became infected in 1987 and earlier. We have some idea that each case costs us about $4,000 for lifetime outpatient care and between $500 and $1,000 per day for hospital management. Therefore, one of the things we can do to reduce costs is to reduce the number of hospital days required by utilizing the best outpatient technology and resources available. And yes, people in the workplace can do a lot to affect these changes by endorsing health-care coverage that reimburses for nontraditional types of patient charges like home health care and outpatient treatment by physical therapists, social workers, mental health counselors, and the variety of other personnel needed to provide quality health-care to people who will most likely die before their fate can be changed.

Likewise, employers must become acquainted with the nature and type of volunteer agencies operating in their communities, and they must both support these groups politically and utilize their resources when appropriate for affected employees. Working to prevent even one case of HIV infection can alter the potential of one life and save our national system hundreds of thousands of dollars in direct and indirect costs.

FEDERAL AND STATE EXPENDITURES

The federal government has been openly and repeatedly criticized for its sluggish and decentralized response to the AIDS issue. In fact, many advocacy groups claim that we would be further along in treatment of the disease and development of a vaccine if a more decisive response had come earlier.

In 1982, only $200,000 was budgeted towards AIDS research, prevention, and control efforts. In the intervening years, millions of dollars were budgeted, and fiscal year 1989's budget had a total request for $1.7 billion for all AIDS-related federal programs. Those federal programs include the United States Public Health Service, the Centers for Disease Control (CDC), medicare and medicaid expenditures related to AIDS, the Department of Defense, and the Federal Bureau of Prisons. Included in this $1.7 billion were millions of dollars earmarked for AIDS-related research that would be administered mostly through the CDC and Health and Human Services divisions of the government.

The Public Health Service has the responsibility for directing monies toward AIDS research and surveillance services. Those surveillance activities are then delegated to the CDC, which have ultimate responsibility for central collection and dissemination of all morbidity and mortality data concerning AIDS-related conditions. The CDC and its administrative superior, the Public Health Service, are also responsible for underwriting test sites all over the country where volunteers can be tested for evidence of infection with HIV under confidential or anonymous conditions.

Another very costly operation at the national level is the mandatory testing of immigrants, federal prisoners, all members of the active duty and reserve forces, and all applicants for military service and the Peace Corps for evidence of infection with HIV. As a small example of costs associated with this program, the testing of just a million military applicants in 1987 cost over $10 million.

Medicare and Medicaid

Medicaid and medicare are forms of federally underwritten health insurance intended for the disabled, the poor, and the elderly. Medicare has not been available to most PWAs because qualifying for benefits takes so long. In fact, only 1 to 3 percent of all PWAs who apply for medicare lives long enough to collect benefits. However, as life expectancy for PWAs increases, more will likely live to receive benefits (McLaughlin, 1988).

Although medicare is entirely underwritten by the federal government (with built-in individual deductibles), medicaid is only partially financed by the federal government, and the rest is covered by state medicaid programs that vary widely from one state to another. In other words, benefits under medicare are equivalent regardless of the state in which one lives, but benefits under medicaid could conceivably be quite different, even in neighboring states.

In the past few years, medicaid has been the means whereby nearly 40 percent of all PWAs paid for their health care, and as many as 80 percent of all PWAs are estimated to become ultimately dependent on medicaid as they deplete personal and family savings and lose private health insurance coverage. The limitations of medicaid provide one of the most important reasons why PWAs should be encouraged to hold on to private health insurance as long as possible.

At this point, most state medicaid programs do not yet have special coverage for AIDS-related conditions, but they are moving toward developing specific written policies. In the meantime, the quality of AIDS-related health care may be at least partially a function of PWAs' state of residence at the time they become symptomatic. For example, although one antiviral drug, azidothymidine (AZT), alone or in combination with other drugs, has been shown to be effective in decreasing the number of life-threatening infections, it is not available to people on medicaid programs in Alabama, Florida, or Arkansas or to unhospitalized PWAs in Wyoming (Buchanan, 1988).

With the cost of AZT currently about $700 per month, the sad reality is that some people dependent on medicaid for health care do not have access to the drug. Speaking strictly from the standpoint of cost, some argue that AZT is too expensive in the long run because it retards the progression of the disease without actually curing it. The end result is that PWAs live longer and therefore potentially utilize more health-care resources than those who live the average AIDS life span of less than two years from diagnosis to death (Buchanan, 1988).

The argument about AZT's benefit in relation to its costs is typical of the kinds of ethical questions raised by AIDS-related diseases that are associated with high death rates. Another health-care-related issue revolves around the hospice movement. Hospice care is a popular concept among patients and health-care professionals alike in this time of concern for human dignity and cost containment.

Clients are typically admitted into hospice care when their medical condition is judged to be terminal. Rather than seeking to prolong life, hospice care is directed at promoting optimal quality of life and death with dignity. The advantages of hospice care are twofold. First, the client can die in a familiar and comfortable environment with ready access to family and friends. Second, hospice care is cost-effective. The actual cost for hospice care directed by a registered nurse who consults as needed with the client's physician is $90 to $140 per day compared to $800 per day for inpatient care. Even so, hospice care is not reimbursed by medicaid in 37 states, although seven of these are reportedly in the process of developing medicaid-reimbursement plans.

State Expenditure on AIDS

Out of necessity, and to augment federal spending, individual and collective state expenditures for AIDS have increased 15-fold between 1984 and 1988, for a total expenditure of $156.3 million in 1988 alone. States not only have to fund their portion of medicaid, but also are responsible for funding state-supervised AIDS counseling and test sites and supporting various educational programs aimed at preventing the spread of AIDS. The states that underwrite AIDS-related activities most heavily are those states that have the most diagnosed cases of AIDS. The five leading states as of late 1988 were California, Florida, Massachusetts, New Jersey, and New York (Rowe & Ryan, 1988).

What is surprising, as well as relatively short-sighted, is the fact that 12 states did not appropriate any monies for AIDS prevention or surveillance. Although these areas have experienced very few cases of AIDS, that no money would be appropriated in the midst of the AIDS epidemic is hard to believe. Legislators and citizens in such states evidently were not listening when CDC representatives stated that AIDS will continue to be concentrated in large cities, but that 80 percent of the growth in new cases by 1991 will occur in areas that are now seeing low incidences of cases (McLaughlin 1988).

CONTRIBUTIONS AND PHILANTHROPY
FROM THE PRIVATE SECTOR

Aside from governmental expenditures related to AIDS, the private sector has contributed untold millions of dollars and human service hours in an attempt to sponsor AIDS-related research, provide direct services to PWAs, and provide prevention-oriented education at the grass-roots level. A partial listing of corporate entities who have found a variety of ways to become constructively involved in some facet of AIDS research, prevention, or control are listed below (AllState Forum on Public Issues, 1988).

- Chevron U.S.A., Inc.
- Metropolitan Life Insurance Company
- New York Life
- USA Life and Health Insurance Group
- Transamerica Insurance Companies
- Times-Mirror Foundation
- Wells-Fargo Foundation
- Levi Strauss Foundation
- Hoffman-LaRoche
- Pacific Mutual Foundation
- Joseph E. Seagram and Sons, Inc.
- Xerox Corporation
- Shaklee Corporation
- Marshall Field, Chicago
- AT&T

In addition to corporate philanthropy, private grant foundations like the Kellogg Foundation and the Robert Wood Johnson Foundation have awarded many grants worth millions of dollars to agencies that provide direct preventive or care services in communities across the country. Volunteer community-based agencies started up in the early 1980s in response to the AIDS epidemic. Some of these organizations, like Gay

Men's Health Crisis (GMHC) in New York City and Shanti Project in San Francisco have grown to national prominence and have annual budgets in the six-figure range. Yet these volunteer agencies are by and large staffed by people who volunteer their time in exchange for an opportunity to help prevent new HIV infections and to care for individuals who have already become infected. Some businesses, small and large, work with these volunteer agencies by grouping together to underwrite the health-care or housing costs of one HIV-infected person, or, to a lesser extent, by providing volunteer groups with office equipment or furniture. Such charitable actions are needed to attempt to address the problems associated with AIDS.

SUMMARY

Health-care costs associated with HIV-related diseases have been discussed as they relate to the health-care delivery system, the insurance industry, the employer, and the public sector. Clearly, as AIDS-related disease becomes more chronic in nature, ambulatory management will have to be a viable alternative to inpatient management if costs are to be minimized.

REFERENCES

Abridge, W. (1988) *Urban/Teaching Hospitals Lose $92 Million on AIDS Patients* (A selected summary of recently published research by grantees of the Robert Wood Johnson Foundation) 2(1):1a.

AllState Forum on Public Issues (1988) *AIDS: Corporate America responds. A report of Corporate Involvement.* New York: AllState Insurance Company.

Buchanan, R. J. (1988) State medicaid coverage of AZT and AIDS-related policies. *American Journal of Public Health* 78(4):432–436.

Eisenstaedt, E. S., & T. E. Getzen (1988) Screening blood donors for HIV antibody: Cost-benefit analysis. *American Journal of Public Health* 78(4): 450–454.

Faden, R. R., & N. E. Kass (1988). Health insurance and AIDS: The status of state regulatory activity. *American Journal of Public Health* 78(4):437–438.

Judson, F. N., & T. M. Vernon, (1988) The impact of AIDS on state and local health departments: Issues and a few answers. *American Journal of Public Health* 78(4):387–393.

Lafferty, W. E., S. G. Hopkins, J. Honey, J. Harwell, P. C. Shoemaker & J. Kobayashi (1988) Hospital charges for people with AIDS in Washington State: Utilization of a statewide hospital discharge data base. *American Journal of Public Health* 78(8):949–952.

Landers, S. J., & G. R. Seage (1988) Medical care of AIDS in New England: Costs and implications. *New England Journal of Public Policy (special issue on AIDS)* 4(1):257–272.

Lipson, B. (1988) A Crisis in insurance. *New England Journal of Public Policy (special issue on AIDS)* 4(1): 285–305.

McLaughlin, L. (1988) AIDS: An overview. *New England Journal of Public Policy (special issue on AIDS)* 4(1):15–34.

Rowe, M. J., & C. C. Ryan (1988) Comparing state-only expenditures for AIDS. *American Journal of Public Health,* 78(4): 424–429.

Scitovsky, A. A., & D. P. Rice (1988) The cost of AIDS care. In K. D. Blanchet, ed., *AIDS: A Health-Care Management Response,* pp. 57–80. Rockville, Maryland: Aspen Publishers, Inc.

Seage, G. R., S. Landers & K. H. Mayer (1988) Medical costs of ambulatory patients with the AIDS-related complex and/or generalized lymphadenopathy syndrome related to HIV infection, 1984–5. *American Journal of Public Health* 78(8):969–972.

3.

FORMULATING COMPANY POLICY REGARDING AIDS

If you ask a manager what the company policy regarding AIDS is, you will most likely be told that the company is concerned about AIDS but has not yet written policies. A national survey of American businesses conducted by Fortune Magazine and Allstate Insurance Company found that 64 percent of the businesses responding were currently concerned about AIDS, but only 10 percent of the companies had written policies (Fortune Magazine & Allstate Insurance, 1988). The fact is that, at best, most companies have some vague notion of how to confront issues regarding AIDS but have not come to grips with how the workplace can develop policies for AIDS. The intent of this chapter is simply to challenge the reader to develop a more definitive company approach to AIDS, which is undeniably one of the most serious health problems of this century.

CORPORATE LEADERSHIP

In a proactive manner, a number of businesses in various parts of the nation have joined forces to address the business impact of AIDS. The Business Leadership Task Force of the San Francisco Bay Area, a coalition of senior managers of corporations in Northern California, organized a one-day symposium and educational materials for use in the workplace. Task force members included Levi Strauss & Co., Pacific Bell, Bank of America, Chevron Corp., Mervyn's, Wells Fargo Bank, and AT&T. With the assistance of the San Francisco AIDS Foundation, this work evolved into a comprehensive package consisting of a 53-page *AIDS in the Workplace* strategy manual for managers and a videotape and brochures for employee education. These materials were produced by the San Francisco AIDS Foundation and are available for purchase (See Appendix E for address).

Another major corporate volunteer effort was the first national conference on AIDS in the workplace held October 13 and 14, 1987, in Chicago. Allstate Insurance Company initiated and sponsored this conference entitled "AIDS: Corporate America Responds." Over 200 representatives from Fortune 500 companies benefited from presentations by U.S. Surgeon General C. Everett Koop, other experts in the field, and from companies reporting first-hand accounts of their experiences with AIDS policy and education. Participants in the conference divided into workgroups and developed position papers on human resources, medical and corporate health services, government and legislative affairs, legal issues, corporate communications, and corporate philanthropy in relation to AIDS (*AIDS: Corporate America Responds, 1988*). The position papers recommended that companies treat AIDS in a manner similar to other catastrophic illnesses, that they refrain from testing for AIDS, and that they do not permit transfers of employees who would rather not work with AIDS patients (Westbrook, 1988).

In an effort to further disseminate such information, "AIDS: A Matter of Corporate Policy," a three-hour, live national video teleconference was presented on May 24, 1988, by PBS National Narrowcast Service in association with the National Lead-

ership Coalition on AIDS and public television station KPBS, San
Diego. Over 3,000 business people in more than 65 localities
participated in this live interactive teleconference. Topics included an overview of AIDS in the workplace; managing the first
case of AIDS; managing health care and employee benefits;
employee communication, education, and assistance; and public relations issues and strategies. As in all of the coalition efforts
thus far, the aim of this conference was to enlighten corporate
America regarding the issues and provide insights into methods
of establishing practical company policies. Resource materials,
including the United Way of America's *Directory of AIDS Re-*
sources (1988) and the American Red Cross pamphlet *AIDS:*
Beyond Fear (1986), were distributed to participants. In addition, the AIDS policy established by U.S. West, Inc., was included in the conference packets.

Major companies have donated countless hours to developing policies regarding AIDS. Employers with AIDS policies include Levi Strauss, Wells Fargo Bank, Pacific Gas and Electric,
University of California, Bank of America, U.S. West, the city of
Alexandria (Virginia), Chevron, Pacific Bell, and AT&T. The information developed can be in turn utilized by large and small
businesses. What are the messages for business in the above
conferences and position papers? First and foremost, more than
20 percent of U.S. companies have already had an employee
with AIDS, and, without a doubt, most companies in this country will likewise experience an employee with AIDS before a
cure is found (Fortune Magazine & Allstate Insurance, 1988).
Second, a significant amount of work has already been done to
develop policies for AIDS, and companies are well advised to
benefit from the experience of other business people and to
develop policies now (Chenoweth, 1988).

WHY DEVELOP AIDS POLICIES?

Businesses in areas with a high incidence of AIDS report from
one to 20 new cases of AIDS each year (Business Leadership
Task Force, 1986). In addition, AIDS strikes most often in the

third decade of life and has a direct financial impact on business (Fruen, 1988). Consequently, companies have become sensitive to the impact of this disease on the individual worker as well as its impact on the quality of work and on fringe benefits such as health-care insurance. Consider the effect of this life-threatening diagnosis on the employee, and the manager can appreciate the need to develop humane, compassionate company policies that help the employee continue to be productive and financially independent. The finding that an employee tests antibody positive (see chapter 4) is not a diagnosis of AIDS; the employee can function effectively for years and can continue to contribute to the job. Companies must anticipate employee concerns about working with an individual with AIDS before an incident occurs. If nothing is done until a situation arises, the suspicion and alarm among coworkers may create walkouts and fear that cannot be abated. At that time even medical information will be distrusted. With early employee education, companies can help prevent the spread of the disease, preserve the dignity of the HIV-infected employee, and ensure a productive work environment and an informed employee population.

Employers who are reticent to develop AIDS policies commonly give the following reasons for not formulating policies in their companies:

1. Developing a policy for AIDS is not necessary because we treat AIDS like other debilitating diseases.
2. A policy may obligate or hold us to something that may be unworkable in the future.
3. Too much uncertainty about the disease and its legal ramifications still exists.
4. Written policy may send a message that we approve of high-risk or morally unacceptable behaviors (*AIDS: Corporate America Responds*, 1988).

Somehow, in the rush to avert policy-making regarding AIDS, the manager with the above reasons has overlooked the need to retain experienced workers and the need to avoid crises that affect production, the bottom line, and the company's reputation. Key reasons for developing an AIDS policy that all managers should scrutinize carefully are as follows:

1. Avoid retraining and hiring expenses by keeping experienced workers on the job, even if AIDS infected.
2. Reduce the possibility of slowed production or walkouts when coworkers oppose working with an AIDS-infected employee.
3. Gain employee respect with a companywide standard approach.
4. Provide support for employees with AIDS by clearly stating policy.
5. Avoid a crisis by anticipating an actual case and being prepared to respond to questions.
6. Earn employee confidence that the company has fully studied the AIDS issue.
7. Review health insurance and benefits plans for adjustments that could control the costs of AIDS health care.
8. Establish policies that comply with legal constraints to avoid employee discrimination suits (Goerth, 1988).
9. Promote a corporate public image that is responsible and caring.
10. Provide employee education programs to help prevent the spread of AIDS (Business Leadership Task Force, 1986).

STRATEGIES TO DEVELOP POLICIES

Given the impetus to develop AIDS policy before the need strikes, how then do we accomplish this work? First and foremost, a task force of key personnel in the company must be identified to complete a plan and implement the effort related to AIDS policy formulation. The task force should be constituted from representatives of the company medical and health unit, senior management, personnel benefits and affirmative action departments, safety, employee assistance, company communications, public relations, legal department, unions, and corporate philanthropy. In addition, anyone with previous experience in managing company AIDS issues, either through past employment or volunteer work, would be a valuable member of the task force.

Leadership on the task force is crucial. Select a leader with the most knowledge about AIDS who also has the ability to organize and complete projects efficiently and thoroughly. One additional criterion for the leader is that this person be able to interact capably with senior management to communicate plans and progress. An initial goal of the task force should be to persuade doubting senior managers that the planning for the policy will be exacting and appropriate to the company's culture and needs. A memo from the chief executive officer directed to all department heads and employees announcing the task force and plans can do much to keep everyone informed that the issues surrounding AIDS will be thoroughly studied.

Second, the task force has to become optimally informed about AIDS and existing employee policies, both within the company and in other companies. As a comprehensive example of an AIDS policy, the Office of Employee Relations, U.S. Office of Personnel Management, issued an AIDS policy bulletin to all federal offices in March 1988. This policy, developed to provide guidance for the public and private sector, addresses the issues of confidentiality, blood donations, and health and safety standards (See Figure 3-1). The full text is included in Appendix B and may be of benefit to a company task force preparing an AIDS policy.

Another guide to developing AIDS policy is the Citizens Commission on AIDS' circular, "Ten Principles for the Workplace." A group of 17 foundations in the New York and northern New Jersey area issued this list in February 1988 to provide leadership as companies consider their AIDS policies (see Figure 3-2).

In addition, members of a company task force need to locate, read, and circulate their trade journals and books with information on AIDS. Experts on AIDS from local and state health

General policy and medical overview
AIDS information and education programs
    Timing and scope of AIDS information and education
        efforts
    Educational vehicles
    Role of the employee assistance program
    Training for managers and supervisors
    Sources of information and educational materials
Personnel management issues and considerations
    Employee's ability to work
    Privacy and confidentiality
    Leave administration
    Changes in work assignment
    Employee conduct
    Insurance
    Disability retirement
    Labor-management relations
    Health and safety standards

Figure 3-1   **COMPONENTS OF THE U.S. OFFICE OF
             PERSONNEL MANAGEMENT AIDS POLICY**
             (see Appendix B for full text)

departments, infectious disease and community health departments in universities, and speakers' bureaus such as the Red
Cross and volunteer AIDS groups ought to be invited to meetings
to provide technical assistance and present facts on AIDS. Task
force members should review the demographics of the workers,
the potential for AIDS in high-risk groups in that geographic
location, and possible hazards in such occupations as laboratory, sanitation, and health-care work, as described in chapter 9.

1. People with AIDS or HIV (Human Immunodeficiency Virus) infection are entitled to the same rights and opportunities as people with other serious or life-threatening illnesses.
2. Employment policies must, at a minimum, comply with federal, state, and local laws and regulations.
3. Employment policies should be based on the scientific and epidemiological evidence that people with AIDS or HIV infection do not pose a risk of transmission of the virus to coworkers through ordinary workplace contact.
4. The highest levels of management and union leadership should unequivocally endorse nondiscriminatory employment policies and educational programs about AIDS.
5. Employers and unions should communicate their support of these policies to workers in simple, clear, and unambiguous terms.
6. Employers should provide employees with sensitive, accurate, and up-to-date education about risk reduction in their personal lives.
7. Employers have a duty to protect the confidentiality of employees' medical information.
8. To prevent work disruption and rejection by coworkers of an employee with AIDS or HIV infection, employers and unions should undertake education for all employees before such an incident occurs and as needed thereafter.
9. Employers should not require HIV screening as part of general pre-employment or workplace physical examinations.
10. In those special occupational settings where there may be a potential risk of exposure to HIV (for example, in health care, where workers may be exposed to blood or blood products), employers should provide specific, ongoing education and training, as well as the necessary equipment, to reinforce appropriate infection control procedures and ensure that they are implemented.

Figure 3-2   **RESPONDING TO AIDS: TEN PRINCIPLES FOR THE WORKPLACE** (Reprinted with permission from the Citizens Commission on AIDS for New York City and Northern New Jersey, New York, NY)

In addition, the task force must analyze existing personnel policies regarding accommodation of an employee with a disability, performance appraisals, hiring and firing, and health benefits. Meeting with insurance representatives may be advisable, to explore benefit packages that would provide optimum coverage for home care to control costs of institutional health care. Another personnel policy to review is that regarding refusal to work or requests for transfers, which would apply in the situation where an employee refuses to work with a person with AIDS. The legal representative on the task force will be instrumental in researching local and state legislation pertaining to legal protection for AIDS patients and federal legislation protecting the disabled. Finally, companies with existing policies and education on AIDS may be consulted for additional advice on how to set reasonable and efficacious policies and programs.

Next, a draft proposal of the policy, including a budget, is to be developed. Assign task force members to write specific components of the policy, and determine deadlines for submission of drafts to the total task force. Necessary components of the policy include a statement of the company's views on AIDS, confidentiality, benefits, reasonable accommodation, testing, and education.

After revising the drafts, the task force should meet with senior management for review, corrections, and approval of the policy. Having an expert on AIDS present at the meeting may be helpful in updating the senior managers on AIDS statistics and answering technical questions. Upon company approval, the task force then should meet with middle management to discuss the company policy regarding AIDS and make plans to utilize inhouse newsletters or bulletin boards to publicize the policy to all employees.

In preparation for dissemination of the company policy, the task force may find reviewing the following self-study questions helpful:

1. What is the company's legal and ethical responsibility toward the employee with AIDS?

2. Will the company's health insurance cover the costs of an employee with AIDS? How will this coverage affect the health insurance costs of the other employees?
3. Will the health insurance or employee assistance program cover the costs of counseling for the employee, family, and coworkers?
4. Will an employee with AIDS be fired or pressured to go on disability? What are the provisions for sick leave, medical leave of absence, and disability?
5. Would the company hire a qualified applicant who is HIV infected?
6. How will a manager respond to an employee with AIDS?
7. Do company managers support the AIDS policy?
8. What plans does the company have for employee education regarding AIDS?
9. What does the company believe about AIDS testing?
10. Will medical information be treated confidentially?
11. Does the health insurance plan provide for case management, AZT and experimental treatment, and home care or hospice care?
12. Will the company honor employee requests for transfer when they do not want to work alongside someone with AIDS?
13. In what ways will a manager assist an employee with AIDS?
14. What job accommodations will be made for an employee with AIDS?

Although these questions are not all-inclusive, they represent the major issues that face an employer. A policy that addresses these issues will create a consistent approach in dealing with AIDS in the workplace.

Evaluation of the policy is the last step in developing AIDS policy. This evaluation will be ongoing as the task force ascertains from middle managers what questions employees are asking. Comments made at educational programs will also be helpful to gauge the reactions of company employees to the policy. The medical, health, and personnel staffs may be able to provide helpful input from their review of the policy and discussions with employees. Periodic update and revision of the policy may be necessary.

COMPONENTS OF AN AIDS POLICY

Four major components of an AIDS policy bear careful scrutiny. In some form, a company planning to write an AIDS policy should include statements related to job accommodation, confidentiality, workplace safety, and testing.

Job Accommodation

Many companies decide to treat employees with AIDS or HIV infection the same as they treat other employees with chronic or terminal diseases and state this in their policy. As long as the employee has no medically prescribed restriction from work, the employee retains employment and all benefits. Most employers subscribe to the view that valued employees should stay on the job as long as their physical condition permits and that a job contributes a measure of security and purpose for the person with AIDS. As expected, complications and concerns surface, however, when the employee with AIDS develops other contagious diseases such as tuberculosis or *Pneumocystis carinii* pneumonia. To cover these cases, employers can include a statement in the policy to the effect that employees have the right to employment as long as they perform the job in a satisfactory manner and do not endanger the health and safety of themselves and coworkers.

Employers are guided in reasonable accommodation by the Federal Rehabilitation Act, which may protect HIV-infected individuals. In this regard, employers review each case individually for job adjustments or reassignments that may help the employee function in the job, given the handicap. The legal obligation for reasonable accommodation does not apply if adjustments would place undue financial or administrative hardship on the employer. Examples of job accommodation include flextime, work at home, more breaks, job sharing, use of labor-saving equipment, and lower salary for reduced job demands (AllState Forum on Public Issues, 1988). No one arrangement may serve an individual with AIDS throughout the period of employment. Flexibility is needed to adjust to the special needs of the employee.

Confidentiality

In effect, the diagnosis of HIV infection obligates an employer to treat this information as confidentially as other medical information; that is, all information pertaining to an employee with AIDS is confidential. A statement regarding confidentiality must be included in the policy. Managers and the medical and nursing staff need to be aware that communicating medical information about an employee to anyone, even the manager's superior, constitutes a breach of confidentiality. Only when the employee grants permission for the information to be disclosed is communicating this information acceptable.

Often a manager becomes concerned about an employee's performance and suspects illness, perhaps AIDS. In these cases, the manager may feel compelled to inquire about the individual's health but is cautioned to ask instead if the company can do anything to help and to provide information about policies for AIDS and other health problems. Likewise, the manager should make no mention of AIDS testing. If the employee volunteers information and does indeed confide in the manager, the manager needs to assure the employee that absolute confidentiality will be maintained.

Rumors present an additional dilemma for the manager. If rumors are circulating that an employee has AIDS, the manager may also become concerned about the health of the individual in question. With this situation, the manager can meet with the employee to offer company assistance, as previously described, rather than to inquire if the rumor is fact. In addition, employees responsible for the rumor are called in to discuss the detrimental effects of this rumor and the company policy regarding AIDS. The manager may ask the medical or employee assistance staff to organize classes, distribute brochures, and arrange counseling sessions for the group to become better informed about AIDS and verbalize their fears.

Workplace Safety

By virtue of the widespread fear of AIDS, companies must take a stand that workplace safety is not jeopardized by working beside someone with AIDS. Because AIDS is not transmitted by casual contact, OSHA workplace safety requirements do not mandate that an employer must notify workers that someone in the company has AIDS (Department of Labor, 1987). The AIDS policy should include a statement referring to the OSHA guidelines (see Appendix D for a full discussion). Although OSHA and the Department of Health and Human Services have initiated a program to ensure compliance with special guidelines for health-care workers, many health-care employers have not fully assumed their responsibility to protect their workers. Professional associations such as the American Public Health Association and the American Occupational Health Nurses Association successfully urged OSHA to develop a formal standard to mandate universal precautions in which all blood and body fluids are treated as though infectious, specify minimum requirements of effectiveness of protective equipment such as gloves, goggles, and fluid-resistant gowns and masks, and require needle-disposal containers made of hard plastic. Recently OSHA announced plans to issue a permanent standard to protect workers from bloodborne diseases.

The company-written policy may also include a medical overview of AIDS. Wells Fargo Bank and Pacific Gas and Electric included such an overview in their policies to explain to employees that AIDS is not transmitted by sharing telephones, office equipment, cafeterias, restrooms, or paperwork but by exchange of body fluids through sexual intercourse, blood transfusion, and intravenous needles and from mother to fetus.

Work disruptions may occur when employees fear working with someone with AIDS. Work refusals and requests for transfer may be anticipated. Coworkers may also resent the special accommodations for an employee with AIDS or feel that the workload has not been distributed equitably. Employers will want to consider including a statement in the AIDS policy that transfers will be granted only in the case of a medical indication for the coworker. Some employers will also ask for volunteers who would want to work in the department with the employee with AIDS so that someone else could be transferred elsewhere. Educational programs on AIDS given by recognized outside authorities may help alleviate some concerns. Group counseling for individuals in a department may help these coworkers cope with the situation and learn to relate compassionately to the individual with AIDS. Moreover, managers should examine the workload in the event that it was not fairly distributed to some employees. If work refusals and slowdowns persist, employers should consult with legal counsel regarding possible disciplinary action.

Family members may also exert pressure on employees to transfer because of their fear that AIDS will be brought home to the family. Educational literature on AIDS can be sent home to families. A monthly newsletter called *Common Sense about AIDS* can be ordered in quantity for employees and families and include a company name on the banner at no extra charge (See Appendix E for address). Another means of providing AIDS information would be for the corporate medical or health staff to have AIDS videotapes available for checkout or to provide special classes for families.

A statement should also be included in the AIDS policy that the company has a vital role in providing health education programs on AIDS. Such a statement directs the occupational health and employee assistance staffs to perform educational activities and supports such duties for these departments. It also informs employees that the company intends to keep everyone up-to-date on AIDS.

Testing

Clearly, AIDS antibody testing at the workplace raises issues of discrimination and invasion of privacy. Most companies are cognizant of the problems that may arise if testing were required for preemployment screening or as a basis for continued employment. These legal issues are more fully discussed in chapter 6.

An employee with undisclosed HIV infection may fear that the employer will require AIDS testing. Most employers include a statement in their AIDS policy to the effect that tests are unnecessary in order to protect the health and safety of other workers because AIDS is not transmitted through casual contact. The Levi Strauss & Co. AIDS policy succinctly states that no AIDS tests will be given to company employees and no questions regarding AIDS will be asked on job applications.

Employees who indicate concern about possible HIV infection and who would like to be tested should be referred to the local health department for information about the location of the nearest federally designated AIDS testing site. All information regarding this request should remain confidential.

Following resolution of the major issues regarding testing, confidentiality, job accommodation, and workplace safety, companies can then examine the need for additional policy statements such as statements on the company's role in AIDS education of employees, managers, and supervisors. In conclusion, all policy statements should be tailored to address the specific concerns and problems that are anticipated for that company.

SUMMARY

To a considerable extent, formulating a company AIDS policy means dealing openly with the issues and setting standards for management decisions. Ultimately, an AIDS policy will yield fair practices for employees with AIDS, ensure smooth operations, and elicit favorable responses from company employees.

REFERENCES

American Red Cross (1986) *AIDS: Beyond Fear* (Available from the American Red Cross, General Supply Division, 7401 Lockport Place, Lorton, VA 22079).

AllState Forum on Public Issues (1988) *AIDS: Corporate America Responds: A Report of Corporate Involvement* New York: Allstate Insurance Co.

Business Leadership Task Force (1986) *AIDS in the Workplace Manual* (Available from the San Francisco AIDS Foundation, 333 Valencia St., 4th Floor, San Francisco, CA 94103).

Chenoweth, D. (1988) AIDS brings new conflicts, employer responsibilities into nation's workplace. *Occupational Safety and Health* 57(7):34.

Department of Labor. (1987) OSHA: Protection Against Occupational Exposure to Hepatitis B Virus (HBV) and Human Immunodeficiency Virus (HIV). *Federal Register* 52(210), October 30, 1987.

Fruen, M. (1988) AIDS: A looming financial commitment. *Business and Health* 5(3):24–27.

Fortune Magazine and Allstate Insurance (1988) *Business Response to AIDS: A National Survey of U.S. Companies*. New York.

Goerth, C. (1988) Restraining order for medical insurance
     urgent attempt to assist AIDS victims. *Occupational
     Health and Safety* 57(7):11.
How companies can ease the burden of AIDS at work (1988)
     Occupational Health and Safety 57(7):12–13, 15–19, 31.
United Way of America (1988) *Directory of AIDS Resources.*
     Alexandria, Virginia.
Westbrook, L. (1988) The corporate community ponders AIDS
     policy. *Business and Health* 5(9):8–9.

4.

SCREENING FOR AIDS

According to Anthony S. Fauci, Director of the Medical Institute of Allergy and Infectious Disease, "There has been no disease in recent memory that has occupied the attention and stimulated the concern of the biomedical community and the lay public as has the Acquired Immunodeficiency Syndrome" (Ungauarski, 1988, p. 20). Some people are prone to point out how little we know about the syndrome, but in reality we have learned a great deal since 1981, when the first cases were reported to the Centers for Disease Control (CDC).

In December 1981, physicians at the CDC debated as to whether AIDS was a communicable disease. It had been reported as a cluster of cases among young white homosexual men who lived in the same geographic vicinity. Therefore, early hypotheses as to the cause of the outbreak included exposure to some common substance such as a recreational

Major portions of this chapter were reproduced from the July 1988 *AAOHN Journal* special issue on AIDS with permisssion of the *American Association of Occupational Health Nurses' Journal* and Slack Publishing Company. The original article, "The Antibody Test for AIDS: Uses and Limitations," was written by Dorothy K. Gauthier and Joan G. Turner.

drug that the men were known to use and an unknown microbe transmitted by some unknown way that was causing some new kind of disease. By mid-1982, investigators at CDC were beginning to see increasing cases of apparently the same disease in blood-transfusion recipients. At that point most hypotheses regarding the disease origin began focusing around a search for the causative microbe (Shilts, 1987).

The first major breakthrough came in 1983 and 1984, when French and American scientists announced that a virus associated with AIDS had been identified. Although the virus was initially given different names, it was renamed human immunodeficiency virus (HIV) by national accord in 1986. Previous to the discovery of HIV, scientists had discovered two other retroviruses associated with human illness, but this virus was clearly different from the earlier two. Since the discovery of HIV, additional retroviruses that cause AIDS-like illnesses have been discovered, and one very similar in character to HIV has been named HIV-2. We will probably come to refer to the original HIV as HIV-1 to differentiate it from subsequent discoveries.

The discovery of HIV as the causative microbe of AIDS was a landmark event for at least two reasons. First, isolation of the virus was accompanied by the promise of a blood test that could serve to signal the presence of the virus in infected individuals. In the absence of a vaccine or specific treatment for AIDS, use of such a test by blood banks would be an important step in helping to eliminate the offending virus from the nation's blood supply. Second, isolation of the virus prompted the United States Public Health Service (PHS) to begin a two-part educational campaign aimed at slowing the spread of the epidemic. By then the virus was thought to be transmitted by sexual contact and blood transfusion, so in May 1983 promiscuous homosexual men were urged by PHS representatives to refrain from donating blood, and they were also warned about the dangers of multiple sex partners. Many viewed the advice as too late because by then a large percentage of gay and bisexual men had already been infected, and the nation's blood supply was also contaminated (Shilts, 1987).

Although not obvious at this point, the virus was already spreading freely among intravenous (IV) drug users in some parts of the country.

ELISA AND WESTERN BLOT TESTS

In May 1985, an AIDS screening test called the *enzyme-linked immunosorbant assay* (ELISA) or *enzyme-linked immunoassay* (EIA) was licensed and released for use in this country. The American Red Cross and other blood banks adopted the test for immediate and sustained use. From initial use of the ELISA in 1985, the American Red Cross announced that nationally, 1 in 500 donors tested positive for the AIDS virus (Shilts, 1987). All infected blood on hand was discarded as would be any future blood found to be HIV contaminated.

Instead of testing directly for the presence of HIV, the ELISA was designed to detect the presence of anti-HIV antibodies, which are formed by the body in response to infection with HIV. This approach was found to be much more reliable and cost-effective than testing directly for the virus; further, scientists knew enough about other infections to realize that a person does not form antibodies until stimulated to do so by bodily invasion with specific microbes.

Not only did blood banks and plasma centers across the nation adopt the ELISA test but also a network of AIDS regional test sites was funded by the CDC for each state in the country. Individual states then decided where these sites should be located so they would be most accessible to potential high-risk populations. These test sites were established so that any concerned person who wanted to be tested could go to the sites and receive confidential testing and educational counseling. The philosophy behind these self-referral centers was that individuals found to be infected with HIV could be counseled to change their behavior to reduce spread of infection.

No laboratory test used in any clinical setting is 99 percent accurate all the time. Even simple blood counts and analysis of body fluids like urine are associated with error; that is, although these tests are usually accurate, mechanical and/or human errors can and do occur. For this reason most physicians repeat tests that are "abnormal" before upsetting patients with potentially erroneous test results.

So the tests developed for screening blood for evidence of HIV infection have a certain degree of predictable error, as do virtually all laboratory tests. To reduce the rate of that error, testing blood for evidence of HIV infection actually requires two tests, the ELISA and the Western blot. The ELISA is comparatively inexpensive (usually less than $10), but it tends to err on the side of "false positive"; in other words, when errors in the ELISA occur, they tend to be those in which the person's blood is actually negative for the anti-HIV antibody, but the test shows a positive result.

To reduce the likelihood of these false-positive results, the following procedure is utilized in screening or testing individual blood samples for evidence of anti-HIV. First, an ELISA is performed. If it is negative, results are reported as negative or nonreactive. If the first ELISA is positive, a second ELISA is performed. If the second ELISA is negative, the individual test results are reported as negative or nonreactive. However, if the second ELISA is also positive, a more expensive confirmatory test ($45 or more), the Western blot (Wb), is performed. When the confirmatory Wb is negative, the individual's test is reported as negative, and the ELISA test results are assumed to have been false positive. When the Wb is positive, however, the individual is considered positive for anti-HIV antibodies and, depending on risk factors, is considered HIV infected.

Why are risk factors like history of blood transfusion, sexual contact with a high-risk partner, or history of hemophilia important? They are important simply because a positive ELISA and Wb in a person with no risk factors associated with HIV infection could represent an overall false-positive test series. Although false-positive results are rare when utilizing the two ELISAs followed by a confirmatory Wb, they do occur. In this instance, a careful evaluation and further testing should be done, probably by a board-certified infectious disease physician.

A few reasons have been offered to explain false positive test results, including: (1) instances in which individuals may have received small doses of noninfectious antibodies in substances such as gamma globulin, (2) the individual may have antibodies *similar* to anti HIV resulting from other past or present autoimmune diseases or viral infections, and (3) procedural errors on the part of clinical laboratory personnel (Coulis & DiSiena, 1987).

What Does a Positive or Negative Test Mean?

Persons who test positive on ELISA and Western blot should always be evaluated for the presence of signs and/or symptoms of AIDS-related diseases. A positive test series, especially in an individual who has had some risk of exposure through sexual contact or blood transfusion or blood products, means that the antibodies to HIV are present in the blood. The individual has been infected with HIV, and the body has subsequently produced antibodies in response to infection. Although the production of specific antibodies is protective or immunizing in some communicable diseases, anti-HIV antibodies do not mean the person is protected against the AIDS virus but means instead that the person is infected with HIV. Such individuals are assumed to have active viral particles in their bodies and are able to pass the virus to others through blood or sexual contact.

Even though the person is infected, a positive antibody test series like the ELISA and Wb does not mean the individual has AIDS. It does mean that the individual has a fairly high chance of developing AIDS-related symptoms (see chapter 1) and of suffering from some AIDS-related disease sometime in the future. No one can predict how long developing symptoms will take, nor definitively say symptoms will occur based solely on these test results.

Conversely, a negative test series means that antibodies to the virus (anti HIV) are not present in the blood. Antibodies may be absent either because the person has not been infected with the virus, or because they have been infected with the virus but have not yet produced antibodies (which takes from two weeks to six months, or sometimes longer). Also, some people who have been in the past (or are currently) engaged in high-risk behaviors such as sexual contact with high-risk people or even recreational IV drug abuse sometimes interpret a negative test result as meaning they have nothing to worry about. Nothing could be further from the truth. Even though the point was made in chapter 1 that every contact or exposure to HIV does not necessarily result in infection, each exposure has the potential to infect, and infections have been documented to have occurred from a single exposure.

BENEFITS AND RISKS OF HIV-ANTIBODY TESTING

Being antibody tested for HIV is a different experience from virtually any other screening test. First, if strict confidentiality is not maintained, the person in question can suffer innumerable personal consequences such as loss of insurance and family upheaval. Typically, ELISA and Wb test results take several days to be reported, and during this time the person tested must deal with a number of psychological issues including the possibility that the test results will be positive.

Another problem associated with antibody testing is that obtaining such testing may have a social stigma attached to it. For example, people in small or close-knit communities are reluctant to seek testing in a centrally located health department setting "because everyone knows me."

These are just a few of the reasons why health professionals are taught to perform a risk-benefit analysis before advising anyone to take the test. During this aptly named procedure, the client and the health professional go over various benefits and risks associated with testing; when potential benefits outweigh identified risks, the individual is then encouraged to be tested. Such testing should be accompanied by appropriate counseling, and confidental results should be given only in person by a qualified counselor who can then help the client understand the meaning and ramifications of the test results.

Benefits of Testing

Possible benefits of testing for the individual include the fact that taking the test and getting negative test results may decrease anxiety in a noninfected person with a low-risk lifestyle. Oddly enough, taking the test and getting positive results can actually act to reduce anxiety in a high-risk individual who may have had some early AIDS-related symptoms but could not be diagnosed until positive test results could be obtained.

Testing may also be beneficial to people who may have had some potential HIV exposure in the past but are now mutually monogamous and want to begin a family. If both partners are negative and have been mutually monogamous for a year or more, they can feel free to begin their family. If either partner tests positive, however, pregnancy should be postponed indefinitely because children born to infected parents have a fifty-fifty chance of being born with AIDS or developing some AIDS-related disease shortly after birth.

When testing is accompanied by good pre- and post-test counseling, another benefit to tested individuals is that they will become more knowledgeable about how HIV is transmitted and how to avoid infection within the constraints of their own personal lifestyle. Additionally, any questions individuals might have about the whole AIDS issue are likely to be answered appropriately by trained professionals.

People other than those tested can also benefit from HIV screening. Through routine screening associated with blood transfusion, for example, HIV-infected blood can be identified and discarded. Additionally, information related to the demographics of persons who are found to be HIV-test positive helps researchers understand more about the prevalence of HIV infection in different segments of the population. Additionally, when demographics like age, race, sex, and geographic locale are analyzed, social researchers can often use the information to design strategies for prevention and control of infection.

Risks Associated with Testing

Risks associated with antibody testing, especially when test results are positive, include depression, anxiety, suicide and sometimes even a desire for revenge. People with antibody-positive test results, whether symptomatic or feeling perfectly well, have a number of important issues to face. Aside from dealing with the ultimate reality of infection with a virus that will affect their potential for health for the rest of their lives, they must decide how to cope with the anxiety generated by that reality. During this process, individuals must also decide who will be told about the situation. For example, all past sexual partners should be notified, and all future sexual partners must be informed.

Another risk for the antibody-positive person is a combination of dread, anxiety, and fear of disease-related symptoms. Understandably, most antibody-positive people are preoccupied to some degree with their individual health status and view with alarm even minor symptoms that may or may not be AIDS related.

Confidentiality or Anonymity?

When antibody testing was started in 1985, the majority of testing was anonymous in nature; that is, the person to be tested gave no name or a deliberate pseudonym and was assigned a random number that would be used when returning for test results. From the standpoint of protecting identity, anonymity was hard to argue against, but anonymous testing does have one danger or limitation. Essentially, if a person tests positive but never returns to get the results (studies show that about 20 percent do not return for results), that individual cannot be reached or urged to return for counseling. For that reason, a growing number of states such as Colorado, Alabama, and South Carolina have changed their public health policies to confidential rather than anonymous testing. When managed conscientiously, confidential testing poses no threat to the customary rights to privacy for the individual.

WHO SHOULD BE TESTED?

In general, and with informed, signed consent and appropriate counseling, the following groups of people should strongly consider being anti-HIV antibody tested:

1. People who have a history (since 1979) of intravenous drug use, especially before they consider pregnancy or elective surgical or dental procedures
2. Sexual partners of drug users and those who have shared any intravenous drug equipment with users
3. Pregnant women who are believed to have a high risk for infection, including those who live in a community where the level of infection, or number of AIDS cases is high
4. Women who seek family planning services should be counseled about AIDS and tested if they have any chance of past sexual or blood exposure to HIV
5. People who have had transfusions of blood or blood components (like plasma) from 1978 to mid-1985 (when blood screening for AIDS antibodies began)
6. Prostitutes or sexually promiscuous individuals
7. Anyone who has had sexual contact with a homosexual or bisexual male in the last ten years

People who have questions about antibody testing, such as who should be tested, where they can be tested, and any other

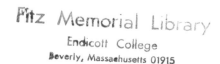

AIDS-related questions should call their local city or county health department or one of the toll-free resource numbers listed in Appendix E.

WHERE TO GO FOR TESTING

When a person has made the decision to be HIV tested, the next question that needs to be answered is *where* they should go for testing among the many good and not-so-good alternatives. The important thing to realize is that a choice exists because most communities offer a variety of places where the test can be done. The most direct way of locating a suitable test site is to call either the local health department or one of the 800 numbers listed in the Appendix E.

Test Sites

The first quality to look for in an appropriate test setting is what measures they take to protect the confidentiality of test results. In fact, calling to ask representatives of the agency to explain the procedures they use to assure confidentiality or anonymity is perfectly acceptable. In ethical settings, a signed consent form, which is congruent with most state laws, may be required. Another quality to look for is that test results should always be given in person, not on the telephone or in the mail. If a fee is charged (and many health department test sites are free of charge), the individual may want to consider ahead of time how to pay. If payment is made with a credit card, personal check, or health-care insurance claim, the individual may, in effect, waive some rights to confidentiality. Rest assured that if the test is billed to a third-party insurer, the fact that the test was done and sometimes even the test results become a permanent part of insurance and medical records.

Another quality of a desirable test site is that trained nurses, health educators, or similarly qualified professionals are present to do one-on-one pre- and post-test counseling. This counseling can be suited to individual needs and time constraints, but at the very least the person tested should have an opportunity to ask questions and should be assisted to begin thinking about how to deal with the test results.

Other questions that should be clarified are how much time should be allowed for the testing, whether any appointment is necessary, and how soon test results will be available. The person being tested should also understand which tests are being used and what their error rate is known to be.

Mass Screening

As has been previously noted, some groups of people in the United States are already being systematically screened for the AIDS virus. These groups include active duty and military reservists as well as applicants to all branches of the military service. If a recruit is found to have evidence of infection, he or she is disqualified for military service for two reasons: (1) the military operates on the assumption that emergency battlefield transfusions may become necessary, and the chances of transfusing HIV-infected blood must be reduced; (2) military personnel are required to take a number of immunizations, including some that could be very detrimental to anyone whose immune system is compromised (which is quite possible in HIV-infected individuals).

Prisoners in our federal correctional institutions have also been undergoing routine AIDS screening. When prisoners are found to have evidence of infection, they are segregated from noninfected prisoners.

Many other forms of mass screening have been and will continue to be suggested. One example is the Louisiana law that requires that all persons applying for marriage licenses submit to AIDS screening. Such programs are unbelievably expensive and fraught with confidentiality and right-to-know problems. Additionally, after spending millions of dollars, the finding is that fewer than one in 10,000 applicants tests positive. Largely because of their overall dissatisfaction with the premarital testing law, many in Louisiana are currently spending more time and money to find a means to repeal the law.

The fact of the matter is that mass screening is not advisable from virtually any standpoint at the present time, and screening operations in the workplace are not recommended under any circumstances. As of 1989, the CDC and other private researchers are doing well-planned random studies across the United States in an effort to ascertain what the rates of HIV infectivity are in various parts of this country. When those studies are completed, we will be better equipped to implement specific prevention and control programs. In the meantime, research efforts to find a treatment that would therapeutically alter the course of infection or even render the infected person uninfected intensify across the country.

SUMMARY

Antibody testing for HIV should never be taken lightly, and HIV screening in the workplace is not recommended. Although the test itself consists of only a small blood sample, the results can alter the way those tested live the rest of their lives. Unfortunately, some undesirables in our society promulgate HIV testing for their own financial gain, and others have no regard for or sensitivity to the necessity for absolute confidentiality. Just as any consumer shops for products or services, individuals are urged to consider alternatives carefully in order to avoid potentially harmful consequences.

REFERENCES

Coulis, P. A., & J. J. DiSiena (1987) AIDS immunodiagnosis: Questions and answers about screening tests. *AIDS Patient Care* 1(1):25–27.

Shilts, R. (1987) *And the Band Played on: Politics, People and the AIDS Epidemic.* New York: St. Martin's Press.
Ungauarski, P. J. (1985) Learning to live with AIDS. *Nursing Mirror* 160(21):20–22.

5.

COMPANY AIDS EDUCATION PROGRAMMING

AIDS has rapidly become one of the most complex public health problems in our nation's history. The U.S. Public Health Service anticipates the total number of AIDS cases will exceed 300,000 by the end of 1991. Yet, as of 1988, only 10 percent of American corporations have developed any policies for dealing with AIDS in the workplace (Kimball, 1988). Although Surgeon General C. Everett Koop noted that educational programs currently in place in American businesses are excellent,

Major portions of this chapter were reproduced from the July 1988 *AAOHN Journal* special issue on AIDS with permission of the *American Association of Occupational Health Nurses' Journal* and Slack Publishing Company. The original article, "AIDS Education at the Worksite," was written by Kenny Williamson, Kathleen Brown, and Joe Packa.

more are needed. Indeed, Dr. Koop has stated that employers have an obligation to provide factual information about the AIDS virus and its transmission.

Even though surveys indicate an increase in public knowledge about the disease, ignorance and misinformation still prevail. For example, many of the same people who report that they understand how AIDS is spread continue to express fear that they or their family members may acquire AIDS through casual contact (American Red Cross, 1987a). As the number of fatalities rises, public fear escalates. Fear can be useful when it helps people change high-risk behaviors, but unreasonable fear can be unnecessarily crippling from the standpoint of workplace productivity and social and emotional health.

How do companies allay these fears and provide employees with the information they need to reduce their risk and simultaneously assist people affected by the epidemic? In the absence of a vaccine, a comprehensive education program is necessary to inform workers in all occupational health settings about AIDS. The federal government has initiated a massive public education effort to provide the American people with factual information on AIDS (Westbrook, 1988). However, coordinated public education efforts have not begun to meet the demand for AIDS-related information; therefore, companies and occupational health professionals must fill the critical need for an educational effort that addresses AIDS risk factors among the general public and in specific occupations at risk. Target groups in the workplace include the estimated one to two million unknowing infected individuals and the worried well who harbor unfounded fears about exposure to the virus. In that education is presently the best weapon against the AIDS virus, many companies have instituted AIDS education programs. The purpose of this chapter is to describe the elements needed for successful AIDS education in the workplace and to identify resources for implementing these programs.

GETTING STARTED

First and foremost, managers must recognize that the threat of HIV infection exists in all companies just as it does in the general population. Some workers are already antibody positive, and some of these will ultimately die from AIDS. Without education among the work group, anxieties, hysteria, and disrupted work routines may result when a worker is found to have AIDS. Unfortunately, in most companies little action has been taken to educate management and employees. During this public health crisis, AIDS education should be considered a primary responsibility of the occupational health unit and should be included as a major topic in each company's overall health education plan.

Because of the sensitive nature of a subject that concerns sexuality and fears of contagion and death, occupational health professionals must be well informed and able to interact with employees about emotion-laden topics. Such concerns may be infrequently addressed in the workplace, and careful planning is needed to develop an AIDS education program that is appropriate and sensitive to the employee population (Baldwin, 1988; Krapfl, 1986). In effect, occupational health professionals must set the tone for the program and communicate with all echelons confidently and without embarrassment relative to the sensitive issues of sexuality and drug abuse. Certainly to be effective educators, occupational health physicians, nurses, and safety specialists must first work through personal feelings about homosexuality, drug abuse, and sexually promiscuous behavior.

As a resource, the occupational health and safety staff collects and interprets the vast amount of information now available about AIDS. Careful scrutiny is needed to ascertain whether the materials are up-to-date and accurate before sharing the information with others in the workplace. By virtue of contacts with the county health department, Red Cross, professional organizations, and other groups concerned with AIDS, occupational health professionals have easy access to an effective network that can provide AIDS education for the occupational health staff during the planning stages (see Figure 5-1).

PLANNING AN AIDS EDUCATIONAL PROGRAM

The best way to respond to the need for AIDS education in the workplace is to develop focused goals or objectives for the program. The goals of AIDS education in the workplace are as follows:

1. To provide employees with reliable, factual information about the risk of AIDS and thus demystify the disease so that behavior changes can be effected to slow the spread of AIDS.
2. To inform and advise management about the nature of the disease and the need for action. Management needs to be informed so as to develop rational, humane policies for both uninfected and infected workers.
3. To prepare the company for the possibility of an antibody-positive person or an AIDS victim among the workforce and thereby avoid reactionary and bitter restrictions and confrontations. Informed managers and workers are likely to give antibody-positive persons support in coping with an uncertain prognosis. Likewise, informed managers and workers will respond to AIDS patients as individuals with a terminal disease who require compassion and full medical benefits.

After formulating goals, the format and strategies for implementing an AIDS education program can be identified (see Figure 5-2). A brief audiovisual presentation or lecture followed by a question-and-answer session is commonly utilized to present AIDS information. Printed literature is also distrib-

1. Acknowledge that AIDS is an essential health education topic for the workplace.
2. Attend professional seminars on AIDS and review professional literature to develop knowledge about AIDS.
3. Contact community resources such as American Red Cross, local health department, and AIDS task forces for educational materials.
4. Identify goals for AIDS health education, for example:
   - To provide employees with factual information
   - To inform and advise management about AIDS
   - To prepare for the possibility of an AIDS case in your company
5. Determine format and educational strategies.
   - Audiovisual presentations. When?
   - Lectures with question-and-answer session. When?
   - Printed materials
   - Company newsletter
   - Posters
6. Offer counseling, education, and referral to those who come to the occupational health unit with questions.
7. Participate in company policy review on issues related to AIDS screening, health benefits, and similar matters.
8. Offer programs and educational materials stressing facts about AIDS.
   - Transmission of the virus
   - Safer sex
   - Special precautions for protecting workers in high-risk occupations
   - Concerns about AIDS testing, the blood supply, co workers with AIDS, and related issues.
9. Evaluate effectiveness of the educational effort through AIDS knowledge and attitude questionnaires.

Figure 5-1 **STEPS IN EDUCATIONAL PROGRAMMING**

TARGET AUDIENCE: 20 male and female employees
                 from the Assembly Department

SCHEDULED TIME: 2:30–3:15 P.M.

OBJECTIVES:
   1. To present facts about transmission of AIDS
   2. To identify high-risk behaviors associated with AIDS
   3. To discuss "safer sex"
   4. To provide an opportunity for participants to discuss
      their concerns about AIDS

STRATEGIES:
   Guest speaker from the American Red Cross
   Distribution of pamphlets *AIDS: The Facts* and
      AIDS, Sex, and You
   Question-and-answer period

EVALUATION AND FUTURE PLANNING:
   Determine the need for additional sessions to discuss
   AIDS topics. These sessions may need to be held monthly
   until all employees have had instruction in facts on transmission, changing high-risk behaviors, working with individuals with AIDS, and company policies regarding AIDS.
   Offer future sessions to update employees on AIDS and to
   reach newly hired employees.

Figure 5-2   **EXAMPLE OF AN AIDS HEALTH
             EDUCATION CLASS**

uted at seminars and can be made available in the occupational health unit. Community speakers' bureaus can usually
provide knowledgeable professionals to speak to company
employees without cost. Another avenue for educating company employees involves the use of the company newsletter to
summarize key information about AIDS prevention.

Not all concerns can be discussed in seminars. As employees come to the occupational health unit, counseling and education should be provided for individuals who express concerns about high-risk behaviors or fears about having been exposed to the AIDS virus. Refer these individuals to the designated testing site nearest your company (usually at a county health department) for confidential screening. Testing at these sites rather than at the worksite is recommended because of the legal issues surrounding screening. In addition, testing sites now provide confidential skilled counseling for medical and social concerns related to AIDS. If you are unable to answer complex questions, have available the telephone numbers of AIDS hotlines or contact testing sites for precise and accurate information.

Developing an AIDS educational program involves review of personnel policies regarding sick leave and medical claims and the local and state laws related to AIDS (de Dios Pozo-Olano, 1987). The likelihood of success in reducing fears depends not only upon providing frank, factual seminars but also upon communicating to employees that management is providing leadership in critically examining all pertinent issues with expert advice rather than prejudice.

Management and employees alike share common concerns and misconceptions about AIDS. The fears are real, and information from all sources must be brought to bear on the concerns. In essence, most employee concerns revolve around two specific issues: (1) Can the company screen employees to identify infected individuals? and (2) How is AIDS contracted? A company AIDS education program must address each of these major concerns.

FACTS ABOUT AIDS SCREENING

Employee screening and the possibility of discrimination against persons with positive tests for the AIDS antibody have produced a legal and ethical controversy that will likely not subside in the near future. An incomplete understanding of the natural history of AIDS virus infection and the nature of the antibody test, known as the ELISA, contribute to the controversy. Currently, several legal and ethical questions regarding AIDS testing in the workplace are being debated. Chief among these are: Can an employer test applicants for AIDS? Can an employer refuse to hire an applicant who admits to having a positive ELISA test? Can an employer require an employee who may have AIDS to be tested? (Klein, 1986). Although all of these questions have not yet been answered, possible solutions may be found by reviewing the laws addressing handicapped and disabled persons. Federal and state laws prohibit discrimination against handicapped or disabled persons. On the federal level, the Vocational Rehabilitation Act of 1973 prevents recipients of federal funds from discriminating against an applicant on the basis of a handicap. Most states also have laws prohibiting such discrimination. The handicapped individual is protected under the law as long as the impairment does not prevent the individual from effectively performing the job; a person who is impaired but otherwise qualified for a position may not be denied or removed from a job and may not be treated differently from other employees in the same position. *People* v. *49 West 12th Street Tenants Corp.* held that AIDS is a protected disability (Creighton, 1986; Williams, 1986).

Based on this finding, the law prohibits employers from asking if an employee has AIDS. An employer may not ask if an applicant is disabled or handicapped unless this disability would substantially interfere with the individual's ability to perform the job. The same principles that prevent an employer from asking about AIDS also preclude testing for the AIDS virus. Indeed, if a suspicion of AIDS is the only reason for testing, then an employer cannot require that the employee have an ELISA performed. If the employee's performance is falling below standard, however, the problem can be dealt with like any other performance problem and a physical examination and/or laboratory testing may be in order.

In summary, testing for AIDS at the workplace appears to be certain to result in job discrimination suits. Corporate attorneys are advising against such screening, and the consensus at a meeting held by the Centers for Disease Control in March 1987 was that "testing violates the public's right of confidentiality, especially because a positive test does not necessarily mean the person will develop AIDS" (The AIDS epidemic and business, 1987, p. 124).

FACTS REGARDING TRANSMISSION OF THE VIRUS

The American Red Cross studied workers in offices, industry, and manufacturing across the state of California (American Red Cross, 1987b). Surprisingly, many common issues and concerns were voiced by employees in all three areas. Primary concerns related to the transmission of the AIDS virus: Can I get AIDS from shaking an infected person's hand? What if I get a paper cut and get infected blood in it? We all share the same bathroom around here...can I get AIDS from using the same toilet as someone with AIDS?

In order to alleviate these fears, employees need to know that AIDS is caused by a virus that cannot be spread by casual, nonsexual contact. AIDS cannot be transmitted through a cough, a sneeze, or a handshake, nor can it be transmitted through food, no matter who prepared and served that food. AIDS is not transmitted by having coffee, going to lunch, or sharing water fountain or toilet facilities with an infected person. The two main ways that the AIDS virus is spread—sexually and through sharing of contaminated needles and syringes among IV drug users—should be stressed. In addition, explain that AIDS has been spread from infected mothers to their newborn infants and by transfusion of infected blood or blood fractions.

All employees should be taught about "safer sex" as a measure to protect themselves from AIDS. *Safer sex* means practicing abstinence or having intercourse only in a mutually monogamous relationship with an uninfected person. When people are not abstinent or mutually monogamous, safer sex methods include appropriate use of condoms as well as body contact without penile penetration (U.S. Department of Health and Human Services, 1987).

Additionally, many workers express fears about the safety of the nation's blood supply. Although the virus has been spread through blood transfusion and blood products in small number of cases (3 percent) the risk of acquiring AIDS in this manner has been greatly reduced. Since 1985, blood collection centers have screened all prospective donors very carefully for the presence of AIDS risk factors and have tested for the presence of the HIV antibody. When the blood tests positive, it is discarded and thus never enters the blood supply. When the HIV antibody or other evidence of infectious disease such as syphilis is detected, blood centers have a further obligation to notify the donor (American Red Cross, 1987a).

The pathophysiology of AIDS is also of concern to workers in all areas. The majority of individuals surveyed correctly stated that AIDS is fatal, but very few could differentiate between HIV infection and AIDS. Therefore, employee education programs should include information on the AIDS virus and its effects. The destruction of the body's immune system and resultant opportunistic infections in persons with AIDS, as well as silent infection with the AIDS virus, should be explained. When discussing asymptomatic antibody-positive individuals, occupational health physicians and nurses should include issues surrounding ELISA testing, such as false positives and false negatives, as well as provide information regarding where testing is available for anyone interested.

Workers with jobs requiring special precautions, such as police personnel, firefighters, emergency medical personnel, and prison employees, may be exposed to blood or body fluids because of accidents, traumatic burn injuries, or violence. For these workers, a few additional guidelines apply (see chapter 9). They must exercise caution to avoid wounds from weapons and punctures from needles used by drug users, use disposable gloves in handling articles contaminated with blood or body secretions, and place contaminated articles in cut-proof evidence bags to be taken to a laboratory for examination or disposal. If a spill occurs, it should be wiped up with a 1:10 bleach solution. Instruct these workers to use an "s-tube" or a hand-operated resuscitator bag if mouth-to-mouth resuscitation is needed (Lansing, 1985).

SUMMARY

If AIDS education programs in the workplace are to be successful, information must be provided by credible personnel with up-to-date, accurate information regarding AIDS and HIV infection. Many resources are available for AIDS education, including union representatives, state or local health departments, and the local chapter of the American Red Cross. Clearly, the best protection we have against AIDS is education. We can no longer afford to hope that AIDS will be defeated before it enters our workplace. As Dr. Koop said, "the day is coming...very soon, when every city, town, every health care institution and provider must deal with AIDS" (Centers for Disease Control, 1985, p. 5). Only through education can companies effectively deal with the threat of AIDS in the workplace and in society at large.

REFERENCES

The AIDS epidemic and business (1987) *Business Week,* March 23, pp. 122–125.

American Red Cross (1987a) *Working beyond Fear.* Los Angeles, California.

American Red Cross (1987b) *AIDS and Your Job: Are There Risks?* Evanston, Illinois.

Baldwin, M. (1988) Education and behavior change in AIDS:
    General concepts. In R. Schinazi & A. Nahmias, eds.,
    *AIDS in Children, Adolescents and Heterosexual
    Adults,* pp. 355–356. New York: Elsevier Publishing Co.
Centers for Disease Control (1985) Recommendations for
    preventing transmission of infection with human T-
    lymphotropic virus type III/lymphadenopathy-associated
    virus in the workplace. *Morbidity and Mortality Weekly
    Report* 34:682–695.
Creighton, H. (1986) Law for the nurse manager: Legal as-
    pects of AIDS. *Nursing Management* 17(11):14–16.
de Dios Pozo-Olano, J. (1987) AIDS education in the
    workplace: Corporate role includes counseling. *Occu-
    pational Health and Safety* 56(13):30–34.
Kimball, M. (1988) *HealthWeek,* February 1, p. 2.
Klein, C. (1986) AIDS and employment issues. *Nurse Practi-
    tioner* 11(5):88–90.
Krapfl, M. (1986) As AIDS hysteria spreads, so does the need
    for cool-headed education. *Occupational Health and
    Safety* 55(4):20–28.
Lansing, L. (1985) HTLV-III exposure during cardiopulmonary
    resuscitation. *New England Journal of Medicine*
    313:1606–1607.
U.S. Department of Health and Human Services (1987)
    *AIDS: Information/education plan to prevent and
    control AIDS in the United States.* Bethesda, Maryland.
Westbrook, L. (1988) The corporate community ponders
    AIDS policy. *Business and Health* 5(9):8–9.
Williams, A. (1986) Public health implications of HIV infec-
    tions. *Nurse Practitioner* 11(10):8–24.

6.

LEGAL ASPECTS OF AIDS AND WORKPLACE DISCRIMINATION

In some societies, any conduct not expressly permitted by the authorities is forbidden. By contrast, in the United States and in any free society, anything not expressly forbidden by law is permitted—and permitted without the need to justify one's actions to the government.

With respect to private employment or access to services, the federal government, through its antidiscrimination laws, expressly forbids a small but important class of conduct. Employers, for example, are generally free to hire and fire whom-

---

This chapter was written by William T. Carlson, Jr., Attorney-at-Law, Haskell Slaughter & Young Professional Association, Birmingham, Alabama.

ever they please, but they cannot lawfully base their decision on certain prohibited criteria, such as race, religion, sex, or, if they receive federal financial assistance, handicap. Any other considerations that an employer might use, whether good or bad, well reasoned or irrational, are simply beyond the scope of these federal laws. They, of course, may be the concern of local laws, private contracts, or economic or social pressure. However, federal and state laws that prohibit discrimination on the basis of handicap are the best vehicles currently in place to address HIV-related discrimination.

THE REHABILITATION ACT OF 1973

Provisions of the Statute

The Federal Rehabilitation Act of 1973 was enacted to govern a wide range of activities relative to the handicapped, including employment. Specifically, Section 504 of the Act prohibits employment discrimination on the basis of handicap by stating that "no otherwise qualified handicapped individual in the United States shall, solely by reason of his handicap, be excluded from the participation in, be denied the benefits of, or be subjected to discrimination under any program or activity receiving federal assistance...." The Act applies to the federal government, federal contractors, and other entities receiving federal financial assistance. Entities receiving federal financial assistance include hospitals, city, county, and state governments, and public schools and universities, among others. Under the Act, such entities may not discriminate against an "otherwise qualified individual with handicaps." In Section 706 a "handicapped individual" is defined as "any person who a) has a physical or mental impairment which substantially limits one or more of such a person's major life activities, b) has a record of such an impairment, or c) is regarded as having such an impairment." Regulations implementing the Act explain that discrimination is prohibited against any employee or applicant "because of any physical or mental handicap in regard to any position for which the employee or applicant for employment is qualified." For example, regulations adopted by the Department of Health and Human Services state that "physical or mental impairment" means any physiological condition or disfigurement affecting a body system or any psychological disorder, mental retardation, and specific learning disability (DHHS Regulations, 1987).

Under the Rehabilitation Act, therefore, an individual must establish that he or she is a *handicapped* individual, that he or she was *excluded* from or discriminated against in a federal or federally funded program, that the discrimination occurred based on the individual's handicap, and that the individual was *otherwise qualified* to participate in the covered program for the Act's antidiscrimination protection to apply (Cooper, 1987). In recent years, the issue arose whether a person with a communicable disease could meet these criteria. In a recent decision, the Supreme Court made clear in *School Board of Nassau County, Florida* v. *Arline* (1987) that a person with a communicable disease can be protected under the Act. Before deciding such a person is eligible for protection, however, courts analyze individual situations to determine whether a significant risk of workplace transmission exists. If a significant risk of workplace transmission exists, the infected individual is not protected from employment discrimination because he or she would not be "otherwise qualified." In other words, a person's handicap must not represent a significant risk to others for the Act's protection to apply. Although *Arline* did not expressly deal with HIV infection, every court that has considered the issue has applied the Supreme Court's analysis in *Arline* to hold that HIV infection is a handicap under the Act. The *Arline* case is illustrative of how a court analyzes cases of persons with communicable diseases, including HIV infection.

The Arline Case

Until the Supreme Court's decision in *Arline* , the most significant opinion on whether HIV infection was a handicap under Section 504 had been a memorandum issued by the U.S. Department of Justice. Charles J. Cooper, the author of the memorandum on behalf of the Justice Department, stated that an employer's fear of contagion removed the protection of the Act for a person with a communicable disease. Furthermore, he stated that persons not suffering any of the disabling effects of AIDS or ARC would have no protection whatsoever against any discrimination resulting from the fact that an individual was seropositive (*Daily Labor Report*, 1986a). The memorandum reasoned that, because these carriers were not afflicted with disabling effects and no physical or mental impairment interfered with any major life function, the carriers were not handicapped under the Rehabilitation Act. The memorandum concluded that employers could take discriminatory actions against persons who were infected with the AIDS virus if they feared that the individual was contagious, even if that fear was irrational.

The Supreme Court's decision in *Arline* was considered by many to be a repudiation of the Justice Department's position. Gene Arline, an elementary school teacher, contracted tuberculosis at the age of 14. Although she was in remission for 20 years, Arline again tested positive for the disease in 1977 and on two later occasions. At the end of the 1978–79 school year, the Nassau County School Board voted to discharge Arline, not because she had done anything wrong, but because of the continued recurrence of the tuberculosis. The trial court dismissed Arline's case after concluding that Congress never intended contagious diseases to be included within the definition of a handicap. However, the U.S. Court of Appeals for the Eleventh Circuit reversed, ruling that diseases are not excluded from coverage under Section 504 simply because they are contagious (*School Board of Nassau County, Florida* v. *Arline, 1985*). As a matter of historical interest, Cooper's memorandum was written between the time of the Eleventh Circuit opinion and the decision of the U.S. Supreme Court. In his memorandum, Cooper labeled the Eleventh Circuit decision "clearly wrong."

By a vote of 7–2, the Supreme Court agreed with the Eleventh Circuit (*School Board of Nassau County, Florida* v. *Arline, 1987*). The vote of the Court is noteworthy because Justice Powell, who voted with the majority, has now retired and Justice Kennedy has taken that seat. Even if Kennedy were to vote for the minority position in a future case, however, such a change would not affect Arline as precedent.

The Supreme Court first concluded that Arline had a "record of an impairment" within the meaning of the Rehabilitation Act because she had been hospitalized for tuberculosis soon after she first contracted the disease in 1957. The Court then rejected the school board's contention, also raised by the Justice Department, that, although she had been impaired, Arline nevertheless was not handicapped within the meaning of Section 504 because her discharge rested on her contagiousness rather than on her diminished physical capabilities. The Court stated specifically, "We do not agree with petitioners that, in defining a handicapped individual under Section 504, the contagious effects of a disease can be meaningfully distinguished from the disease's physical effects on a claimant in a case such as this. Arline's contagiousness and her physical impairment each resulted from the same underlying condition, tuberculosis. It would be unfair to allow an employer to seize upon the distinction between the effects of a disease on others and the effects of a disease on a patient and use that distinction to justify discriminatory treatment" (*School Board of Nassau County, Florida* v. *Arline, 1987*, p. 1128). The Court concluded that Congress intended to protect persons with impairments that "might not diminish a person's physical or mental capabilities, but could nevertheless substantially limit that person's ability to work as a result of the negative reactions of others to the impairment." (*School Board of Nassau County, Florida* v. *Arline, 1987*, p. 1129). In a footnote, the Court noted that it was not deciding the issue of whether HIV-infected people are protected under the Rehabilitation Act because the case before it concerned tuberculosis. Both before and after the Supreme Court's decision in Arline, however, lower courts have held that people with AIDS, as well as those infected with HIV, are covered as individuals with handicaps under Section 504. These cases were *Chalk* v. *Orange County Department of Education* (1988) and *Thomas* v. *Atascadero*, (1987).

However, a finding that a person is handicapped is only half of the determination necessary before applying the protection of Section 504. The individual must also be "otherwise qualified."

The "Otherwise Qualified" Requirement

The fact that people with contagious diseases are protected under the Rehabilitation Act does not mean that an employer must disregard the fact that an applicant or current employee has a contagious disease. Section 504 requires that an individual be "otherwise qualified" for a particular position or program. "An otherwise qualified person is one who is able to meet all of a program's requirements in spite of his handicap" (*Southeastern Community College* v. *Davis*, 1979). To be "otherwise qualified," individuals with a contagious disease must not pose a significant risk of transmitting the disease to others. If such a risk exists and cannot be eliminated by reasonable accommodation, then that person is not "otherwise qualified" under the Act and therefore is not protected in the particular job. In the employment context, an otherwise qualified person is one who can perform "the essential functions" of the job in question. Recently Congress amended the Rehabilitation Act to make this clear (Federal Regulations, 1987).

In the Civil Rights Restoration Act of 1988 (P. L. 100-259), which was passed by both houses over the president's veto on March 22, 1988, Congress added a provision regarding individuals with contagious diseases and infections. This provision states that, for purposes of Section 504, the term *individual with handicaps* does not include an individual who has a currently contagious disease or infection and who would constitute a direct threat to the health or safety of other individuals or who is unable to perform the duties of the job because of the disease or infection. The Congressional amendment closely parallels the guidelines set forth by the Supreme Court in *Arline*. The Court suggested that an employer would have to make the "otherwise qualified" decision based on a case-by-case review of the facts. Based on a suggestion from the American Medical Association, the Court stated that the following facts should be considered in determining whether the contagious nature of the handicap disqualifies an individual from a job:

1. The nature of the risk (how the disease is transmitted)
2. The duration of the risk (how long the carrier is infectious)
3. The severity of the risk (the potential harm to third parties)
4. The probabilities that the disease will be transmitted and will cause varying degrees of harm

The Court did not state the level of proof an employer must have to disqualify an individual because of his or her contagious disease. However, the Court stated that deference should be given "to the reasonable medical judgment of public health officials" (*School Board of Nassau County of Florida* v. *Arline, 1987*, p. 1131 n.18). This can be interpreted as a signal from the Court of its willingness to accept the recommendations of the Centers for Disease Control in this area. Note that the Court did not decide whether an employer could rely on advice given by a private physician.

Again, "otherwise qualified" means that an individual does not represent a danger of contagion to others and is able to perform the duties of the position for which he or she is to be employed. When the progress of a disease has reached the point where the employee can no longer perform the substantial activities of the position, that employee is not otherwise qualified, and the Rehabilitation Act does not require that the employer maintain that employee on the payroll. However, employers are required to treat all employees comparably who have ceased to be able to work due to medical conditions. In other words, an employer's policy concerning medical or other disability is equally applicable to persons with AIDS.

The "Reasonable Accommodation" Requirement

The Supreme Court has held that the Rehabilitation Act requires an employer to provide reasonable accommodation for handicapped workers (*Southeastern Community College* v. *Davis*, 1979; Federal Regulations, 1987). The purpose of the reasonable accommodation requirement is to allow a handicapped person to become "otherwise qualified" for a particular position. Reasonable accommodation in the HIV context might encompass flexibility regarding working hours, time off for medical visits and treatment, and some restructuring of job duties.

Given the facts of a particular situation, the employer might within the definition of reasonable accommodation reassign an individual's job duties if such action is justified by the individual's condition. However, an employer probably cannot take such an action, even without compensation reduction, in order to deal with the anxiety of coworkers or customers. In *Chalk* v. *Orange County Department of Education* (1988), the school board reassigned a classroom teacher with AIDS to an administrative position coordinating grant applications. Chalk asked the federal district court for a temporary injunction ordering the county to return him to the classroom because he feared he might not survive until the trial, but the court refused. The U.S. Court of Appeals for the Ninth Circuit in San Francisco reversed the district court and granted an injunction placing Chalk back in the classroom. The appeals court held that the overwhelming consensus of medical opinion supported the conclusion that the teacher could not transmit his disease on the job, and the fear of parents concerning the teacher's disease was not sufficient reason to remove the teacher from the classroom.

The employer's only duty is to make a reasonable accommodation for the employee's or potential employee's handicap. If the making of the accommodation would result in an "undue financial or administrative burden" on the business or would require a fundamental alteration in the nature of an activity, no accommodation is required (*Southeastern Community College v. Davis*, 1979, pp. 2368, 2370). Neither does the law require fruitless accommodation, where the employer's assistance would not overcome the effects of a person's handicap (*Alexander* v. *Choate*, 1985). In such a case, the employer is not required to find another job for an employee who is not qualified for the job he or she was doing or has applied for, but the employer cannot deny such a person alternative employment opportunities reasonably available under the employer's existing policies (Federal Regulations, 1987).

NATIONAL LABOR RELATIONS ACT

Section 8(d) of the National Labor Relations Act (1935) requires that the employer and union bargain "in good faith" with respect to wages, hours, and other terms and conditions of employment. Safety rules and practices are considered to be "conditions of employment" under this section, as was decided in *NLRB* v. *Gulf Power Company* (1967). A union could conceivably claim that an employer has a duty to bargain over any proposed AIDS policy or testing program if the employer suggests such a policy is safety related, especially if it covers current employees who are unionized.

If AIDS issues are a subject of mandatory bargaining, other issues arise regarding the flow of information between the employer and the union. The employer's duty to bargain in good faith includes an additional duty to supply the union with "requested" information that will enable the union to negotiate effectively and to perform properly its other duties as bargaining representative (*Local 13, Detroit Newspaper Printing and Graphic Communications Union* v. *NLRB*, 1979). At some point, a union may demand information pertaining to the health of an employee or employees suspected of being infected with the AIDS virus or who is symptomatic for one of the diseases related to AIDS. An employer should vigorously resist providing such information to a union because the HIV status of any employee would be irrelevant in most cases, especially to determine the propriety of a corporate AIDS policy or testing program.

Indeed, this position has case support. In *Oil, Chemical and Atomic Workers Local Union #6-418* v. *NLRB* (1983), the union contended that, in order to bargain effectively on issues pertaining to health and safety, it needed various company health and safety records, including worker mortality statistics, laboratory studies of employees, and health information obtained through workers compensation and insurance claims. Although the company objected to the release of the information, the court held that if the employer could delete from the records any other information that could link the record to a specific employee, releasing the information would not violate employee rights to privacy and confidentiality. If the information provided could not be traced to the identity of an individual employee, the release of information would be acceptable. This decision assumes, of course, that the workplace is sufficiently large and that the employee's identity could not be determined as a matter of deduction.

Another section of the National Labor Relations Act, Section 157, gives workers the right "to engage in ...concerted activities for the purpose of ...mutual aid or protection." Both union and nonunion employees may be protected when they protest what they in "good faith reasonably believe" to be an unsafe working condition. A case example was *NLRB* v. *City Disposal Systems, Inc.,* (1984). If an employee were to oppose the employment of an individual with AIDS or refuse to perform services for a person with AIDS because doing so was "unsafe" and the employer acceded to the demands of the employee, the employer would conceivably claim to be acting in accordance with the National Labor Relations Act. The National Labor Relations Board, the federal administrative body that interprets the Act, has not expressly addressed this issue, but given current medical information concerning workplace exposure, the Board would be highly unlikely to find that the employer acted on a "reasonable and honest belief." One commentator at the American Bar Association annual meeting on August 10, 1986, suggested that workers could use the "fear of contagion" exception created by the Justice Department memorandum on Section 504 to justify their "honest belief." However, the Arline decision probably was effective in nullifying such an assertion (Daily Labor Report, 1986b).

OCCUPATIONAL SAFETY AND HEALTH STANDARDS AND APPLICATION

Under the federal Occupational Safety and Health Act of 1970 (OSHA, 1970), employers generally have two duties as stipulated in Section 654: a specific duty to comply with all occupational safety and health standards promulgated by the government and a general duty to furnish employment in a workplace "free from recognized hazards that are causing or are likely to cause death or serious physical harm...." This second statutory clause is OSHA's "general duty" clause. In Section 660 (c)(1) OSHA also prohibits employers from retaliating against employees who refuse to be exposed to a health hazard that they have asked the employer to correct and that they in good faith reasonably believe poses a danger of death or serious injury.

In July 1987, OSHA announced an action plan to protect health-care workers from exposure to hepatitis B and AIDS. OSHA stated that it would rely on the general duty clause of the Occupational Safety and Health Act to enforce compliance with CDC guidelines concerning protection of health-care workers while it developed its own rules as an administrative agency. The Centers for Disease Control (CDC) issued its most comprehensive guidelines in its *Morbidity and Mortality Weekly Report* (1987), and these still serve as the basis of OSHA-mandated protection guidelines.

Later in 1987 OSHA issued regulations categorizing the risks that health-care workers faced in various patient-care activities. The purpose of these regulations was to give hospitals and their employees an idea of how to categorize the risk of HIV transmission posed by various job-related tasks and, thereby, the extent to which universal barrier precautions should be utilized. For example, handling of patient utensils and noninvasive touching of patients are considered Category III tasks and require little or no protective guard. However, procedures that involve an inherent potential for spills or splashes of blood or other body fluids are Category I tasks, and appropriate protective clothing and measures are required.

Finally, in January 1988, OSHA issued an inspection policy for health-care facilities (DOL/OSHA, 1988). Again utilizing the general duty clause, OSHA announced that it would inspect facilities to ensure that universal precautions were in use by employees. The OSHA regulations also stated that the agency had identified the states with the largest number of AIDS cases and that inspection of health-care facilities in those states would be in greater proportion than inspections in states with few AIDS cases. Therefore, Florida and New York hospitals have received more inspections than those in Alabama and South Dakota, for example. However, an inspection that disclosed a failure to follow universal precautions could result in a fine of $10,000 against the facility, regardless of where the facility is located.

OSHA and Employee Refusal to Treat or Assist

Employers must recognize that they may occasionally have an employee who refuses to work with a coemployee who is HIV infected or to treat or assist an AIDS patient or other type of client. To avoid employee claims that they have a good faith reason to believe that a fellow employee or client poses a danger of death or serious injury, employers have the affirmative responsibility to educate their employees concerning workplace transmission. After providing education to the employee(s), if an employee simply refuses to perform his or her duties in relation to HIV-infected persons, the issue becomes a legal and administrative problem to be resolved on an individual basis. However, OSHA is unlikely to be a barrier to the termination of such an employee. Before making such a termination decision, the employer should investigate the basis for the employee's refusal to work to ascertain that the refusal is based on irrational fear. If the employee has some physical condition that places the employee at greater risk for HIV transmission, the employer has an affirmative obligation to separate that employee from the potential risk. In most cases, this greater risk will not be present and the employer should follow whatever guidelines it uses in dealing with such cases where no risk of contagion exists.

EMPLOYEE RETIREMENT INCOME SECURITY ACT (ERISA)

The Employee Retirement Income Security Act (ERISA) was enacted in 1974 to set standards for employee benefit programs and to protect employees from actions taken based on their eligibility for benefits. Specifically, Section 510 of ERISA prohibits employer action against current employees to deprive them of benefits under ERISA-protected plans. Health insurance is included as an employee benefit program covered by ERISA. Unlike the handicap discrimination laws, which do not apply universally, ERISA applies to all employers who maintain employee benefit plans. Consequently, an employer who is not otherwise prohibited from engaging in HIV-related discrimination may be prohibited from terminating a current HIV-positive employee for the purpose of avoiding medical care costs.

One federal court has applied ERISA in this manner (*Folz* v. *Marriott Corp.*, 1984). An employee of a large hotel chain learned he had multiple sclerosis and told his employer. A few months later he was fired. A Missouri federal court held that the termination was improperly motivated by the company's desire to avoid additional expenses to its health insurance plan and thus violated section 510 of ERISA. The court ordered the employee reinstated with back pay and payment of benefits lost due to the termination.

STATE AND LOCAL LAWS

A number of states and municipalities, for example, Wisconsin and the District of Columbia, prohibit discrimination on the basis of sexual orientation. Exclusion of all persons who are, or are perceived to be, at high risk for HIV infection will probably violate such laws. In addition, virtually all jurisdictions prohibiting discrimination on account of sexual orientation also have laws prohibiting handicap discrimination, thus providing a second basis for potential liability against those who discriminate against HIV-infected persons in those jurisdictions.

A greater number of states have handicap discrimination laws than have sexual orientation laws. Although not all persons in high-risk groups have HIV, a member of a high-risk group excluded from a job may have a plausible claim if he or she can prove that the discrimination occurred because he or she was perceived to be infected or at risk for infection. In other words, this person would be perceived as handicapped (Federal Rehabilitation Act, 1973). Discrimination based on this *perceived* handicap would represent a cognizable basis for a claim under federal and most state handicap laws. However, the affected person must prove that the discrimination was not based solely on sexual orientation, but rather on the perception that a handicap exists because the individual is at risk for HIV infection.

Issues of unemployment compensation also must be considered. Employees who voluntarily resign from their positions must prove they had good cause to quit and that they are able and available for other employment before they can receive unemployment benefits (National Foundation, 1985). Good cause is necessarily a relative term because states differ in their interpretation of the phrase. Some states consider any employee illness good cause for a voluntary resignation, but most restrict good cause to work-related illnesses (*Duffy* v. *Labor and Industrial Relations Commission*, 1977). In those states, persons with AIDS who are forced to quit due to illness would not qualify for benefits because the disease is not work related unless, of course, they could establish that they were exposed to it at work. Moreover, even if the illness were connected to employment, individuals with AIDS still would be denied benefits in most states if they are not available to perform other suitable work that might be offered. For example, in *Carter* v. *Unemployment Compensation Board of Review* (1982) the court's decision was that the claimant must be able to work and be available for suitable work in order to be entitled to benefits. Unemployment compensation is not health insurance, and it does not cover the physically or mentally ill during the periods they were unemployable. For those who leave work due to harassment, however, unemployment benefits could be available under theories of constructive discharge or because of resignation for good cause: for example, in *Richards* v. *Daniels* (1981) a teacher voluntarily quit with good cause after being mistreated by other teachers and the principal when she refused to sign a petition.

Employers also have alternatives. Most companies and businesses have leave-of-absence policies that contemplate long-term illness, and diseases associated with AIDS should be covered by such policies. Some employers also have long-term disability plans that would cover persons with AIDS. Also, a business may wish to place such employees in noncritical positions so that they could maintain their jobs even if they missed workdays due to illness. In all of these matters, the employer and the affected employee should discuss the issue completely before any action is taken.

TESTING FOR THE HUMAN IMMUNODEFICIENCY VIRUS

In examining the broad spectrum of AIDS-related legal issues, the most sharply debated is probably the right of employers or others to test individuals for HIV. A number of legal considerations should be part of any decision-making process concerning this issue.

Some states and localities have enacted legislation banning AIDS testing or limiting the use of test results in the employment context. For example, a California law, effective January 1, 1986, bans the use of test results for the AIDS virus "for the termination of maturability or suitability for employment (*Labor Relations Reporter*, 1986). In Massachusetts the Commission against Discrimination stated that preemployment inquiries concerning AIDS are prohibited (*Employment Practice Guide*, 1986a). The New Jersey Division of Civil Rights announced that state law prohibits an employer from conditioning employment on taking an AIDS test unless the employer can show that an employee who tests positive could not perform the job in question without jeopardizing the health and safety of the employer or others (*Employment Practice Guide*, 1986b). The mayor of Philadelphia, W. Wilson Goode, issued an executive order prohibiting the screening of city employees or clients for AIDS (*Daily Labor Report*, 1986c). Last, Section 3809 of San Francisco Ordinance N. 49985 prohibits testing designed to show that a person has AIDS or any AIDS-associated condition unless the employer "can show that absence of AIDS is a bonafide occupational qualification" (*Employment Practice Guide*, 1985). Even without specific legislation, employers may be prohibited from using the results of such tests for employment decisions in jurisdictions in which AIDS is a protected handicap. Under most handicap discrimination statutes, employers may consider AIDS test results in employment decisions only if they can show a link between test results and job qualification. In other words, unless the employer could prove that persons testing positive for AIDS antibodies are not "otherwise qualified" for the job, the use of test results as an exclusionary standard would be prohibited (Federal Regulations, 1987). A situation in which an employer could establish that the presence of HIV in an employee's blood would cause that person to become unable to perform a given job would be unusual.

In addition to statutory restrictions on the right to screen for AIDS, most states recognize a general right to personal privacy. This right protects an individual from unreasonable intrusion into their private affairs. In the employment context, such suits involve the employer's accumulation of "private information," such as the accumulation of unnecessary personal or medical information. An actual intrusion might occur if an employer performed an AIDS test without the employee's knowledge or consent. The intrusion "must be something which would be offensive or objectionable to a reasonable person" (Keeton & Prosser, 1984). To many people, the use of a blood sample for an AIDS test without consent would be considered unreasonable and objectionable. Before imposing liability, however, courts balance the employer's need to know the accumulated information against the employee's reasonable expectation of privacy; for instance in *Simmons* v. *Southwestern Bell Telephone Company* (1978), the employee was held to have no reasonable expectation of privacy in personal telephone calls made from a telephone he knew would be monitored.

Medical tests, including tests for AIDS, might run afoul of public employees' Fourth Amendment right to privacy and to be free from unreasonable searches and seizures. In *Caruso* v. *Ward* (1986) the court struck down a random drug-testing policy because the policy did not meet the reasonableness requirements of the Fourth Amendment. Given the current position of the Centers for Disease Control that AIDS is not transmitted by casual workplace conduct, but only by conduct of an intimate nature, employers may have difficulty establishing that they need to know if an applicant is positive for the AIDS antibody. Nevertheless, at least two federal agencies have begun AIDS-testing programs for employees and applicants because of job-specific criteria. The State Department tests all foreign service applicants, employees, and their dependents because of the lack of high-quality medical services in some job situations and the documented need of the State Department to use its foreign service employees for blood donations (*Daily Labor Report*, 1986d). The Department of Labor also conducts AIDS tests on job corps applicants and current trainees on the basis of its responsibilities for the health and safety of corps members who live in residential centers (*Daily Labor Report*, 1986e). In another case in which a state employer attempted to test public employees for HIV, however, federal courts have struck down the testing program as violative of the Fourth Amendment (*Glover* v. *Eastern Nebraska Community Office*, 1988).

In addition, federal regulations (1987) issued pursuant to Section 504 of the Rehabilitation Act of 1973 prohibit such testing. Under Section 84.14(a) of the regulations, an employer may not conduct any type of preemployment medical examination or testing unless it is job related. An employer covered by the Rehabilitation Act could not, therefore, require that an individual be tested for HIV unless that inquiry could be shown to be job related. This does not rule out the use of preemployment physicals by employers. If HIV testing is part of the preemployment physical given to all potential employees, such testing is permitted. However, the results of the test can be used only in accordance with the requirements stipulated in Section 84.14(c) of the regulations. In other words, an employer would be unable to discriminate against a potential employee on the basis of the HIV test results alone.

To the extent that employers may be concerned that a failure to test may render them liable to other employees or customers, a federal court decision in Washington, D.C., suggested that adherence to CDC guidelines may bar such claims. In *Cozup* v. *Georgetown University* (1987), a federal court granted judgment in favor of a hospital and blood bank that provided HIV-tainted blood transfusions to a premature infant. The court stated that the agencies followed the procedures dictated by the medical information available at the time of the incident and therefore were not liable in this case.

SUMMARY

At this time, federal and state laws and regulations prohibiting discrimination of handicapped persons are the basis for addressing HIV-related discrimination. Issues regarding employee refusal to work with someone with AIDS, job accommodation and health benefits for the HIV-infected employee, and AIDS testing were covered in this chapter. In all these situations, employers and employees should discuss the issues completely before any action is taken.

REFERENCES

Alexander v. *Choate*, 105 S. Ct. 712, 720, and n.19 (1985).

Carter v. *Unemployment Compensation Board of Review*, 442 A.2d 445 (1982).

Caruso v. *Ward*, 506 N.Y.S. 2d 789 (1986).

Chalk v. *Orange County Department of Education*, 840 F.2d 701,711 (9th Cir. 1988).

Cooper, C. J. (1987) Discrimination against the handicapped. In W. Dornette, ed., *AIDS and the Law*, pp. 141–147. New York: John Wiley.

Cozup v. *Georgetown University* 663 F. Supp. 1048 (D.C.) 1987.

Daily Labor Report (BNA) No. 122, D-1, D-8, D-12 (June 25, 1986a).

Daily Labor Report (BNA) No. 156, A-8 (August 13, 1986b).

Daily Labor Report (BNA) No. 86, A-4 (May 5, 1986c).

Daily Labor Report (BNA) No. 231, A-9 (December 2, 1986d).

Daily Labor Report (BNA) No. 244, A-2 (December 19, 1986e).

Department of Health and Human Services Regulations, 45 C.F.R., Section 84.3 (j) (2) (i) (1987).

DOL/OSHA. Enforcement procedures for occupational exposure to blood-borne infectious agents in healthcare facilities. OSHA Instruction CPL 2-2-44. U.S. Department of Labor (January 19, 1988).

Duffy v. *Labor and Industrial Relations Commission*, 556 S.W. 2d 195 (Mo. Ct. App. 1977).

Employment Practices Guide 2 (CCH) paragraph 5025 (January, 1986a).

Employment Practices Guide 2 (CCH) paragraph 5027 (January, 1986b).

Employment Practices Guide 5 (68) paragraph 20, 950 (B) (December, 1985).

ERISA, 29 U.S.C. Section 1140, 1974.

Federal Regulations of the Rehabilitation Act, 45 CFR, Section 84.3, 84.12 (K) (1987).

Federal Rehabilitation Act of 1973, Sections 504, 706 (7)(b), 794.

Folz v. *Marriott Corp.*, 594 F. Supp 107 (W.D.Mo. 1984).

Glover v. *Eastern Nebraska Community Office*, 46 *Employment Practices Guide* (CCH) Paragraph 37,909 51, 727 (D.Neb. March 29, 1988).

Keeton, R., & Prosser, W. (1984) *Law of torts* (5th ed.). St. Paul: West Publishing Co.

Labor Relations Reporter 4 (BNA) 14:210 (h)(September 29, 1986).

Local 13, Detroit Newspaper Printing and Graphics Communications Union v. NLRB, 598 F.2d 267,271 (D.C. Cir. 1979).

Morbidity and Mortality Weekly Report, 36 (2s) (August 21, 1987).

National Foundation for Unemployment Compensation and Worker's Compensation (January 1985) *Highlights of State Unemployment Compensation Laws*, 3.

National Labor Relations Act, 29 U.S.C. Section 158(d) (1935).

NLRB v. *City Disposa-+l Systems, Inc.*, 465 U.S. 822, 837 (1984)

NLRB v. *Gulf Power Company*, 384 Fed. 22, 825 (5th Cir. 1967).

Oil, Chemical and Atomic Workers Local Union # 6–418 v. *NLRB*, 711 F.2d 348, 352-57, 363 (D.C. Cir. 1983).

OSHA, 29 U.S.C. Sections 651-678 (1970).

OSHA Regulations, 52 Fed. Reg. 41821 (October 30, 1987).

Richards v. *Daniels*, 615 S.W. 2d 399 (Ark. 1981).

School Board of Nassau County, Florida v. *Arline*, 772 F.2d 759, 764 (11th Cir., 1985).

School Board of Nassau County, Florida v. *Arline*, 107 S. Ct. 1123-31 (1987).

School Board of Nassau County, Florida v. *Arline*, 29 U.S.C. Section 706 (7)(B)(ii)(1987).

Simmons v. *Southwestern Bell Telephone Company*, 452 F. Supp. 392 (W.D. Okla 1978).

Southeastern Community College v. *Davis*, 99 S. Ct. 2361, 2367-70, (1979).

Thomas v. *Atascadero Unified School District*, 662 F. Supp. 376, C.D. Cal., (1987).

7.

WORKERS' FEARS ABOUT AIDS

As AIDS infects more individuals in this country, the number, circumstances, and hardships of having company personnel with AIDS will increase. Because most individuals with AIDS are in their young adult years, AIDS will have an unrelenting impact on our work setting. Indeed, by some projections, AIDS may become the number one source of death in this age group by 1991 (Quinn, 1987). No wonder fear of AIDS has escalated in most work settings and in the general public.

Our ignorance of AIDS shows up in the fears which people exhibit as they try to come to grips with the disease. In the work setting, this fear can generate severe negative behaviors such as ostracism of the coworker with AIDS, anger, and walkouts. The

---

Major portions of this chapter were reproduced from the July 1988 *AAOHN Journal* special issue on AIDS with permission of the *American Association of Occupational Health Nurses Journal* and Slack Publishing Company. The original article, "Workers with AIDS: Attitudes of Fellow Employees," was written by Beverly Hansen, Wendy Booth, Hala Fawal, and Rebecca W. Langner.

purpose of this chapter is to examine the sources of these fears and to recommend strategies for combating fear in the workplace.

HYSTERIA AND PANIC

How, then, do we explain the fear and manifested hysteria? One apparent source of fear is the media's sensationalization of AIDS. "Exaggerated media reports that distort factual assertions and medical evidence" have been widespread (Business Leadership Task Force, 1986, p. 4). The public is dependent on the media for information; conflicting reports and misinformation have been rampant. Thus, ever-present news reports have hastily presented one sensational story after another and generated escalating fears along the way.

Another source of fear about AIDS can be attributed to a generation of young and middle-aged adults lacking experience with widespread epidemics of polio, tuberculosis, and pneumonia. American citizens thought that infectious disease epidemics happened in the past, not today. For the most part, during our lifetimes infectious diseases have been controlled with medications or vaccines. Now, a fatal, little-known infectious disease is spreading unchecked without cure in our society.

Additional fears have been generated by reports that unsuspecting individuals contract the disease. Persons who received blood or blood products, women who did not know their husbands were bisexual, and newborn babies of mothers who are drug users have all been infected with AIDS. Police officers, health-care workers, prison guards, and sanitation workers are becoming increasingly concerned about the occupational hazards of acquiring the disease because of their contacts with HIV-infected individuals. The psychological effects of having to work with AIDS cases and the precautions necessary to be protected from individuals with unknown status appear in professional and trade journals as well as the popular press (Turner et al., 1988). We are afraid for ourselves and our children.

EMOTIONAL REACTIONS

Four types of emotional reactions arise directly from concerns about this mysterious disease and the cultural taboos regarding sexuality and death and dying. These reactions include:

1. Fear of contagion
2. Homophobia and fears associated with other lifestyle behaviors
3. Overidentification
4. Fear of death and dying

Fear of Contagion

Conjecture about the nature of AIDS and early uncertainty about modes of transmission have contributed to a fear of contagion. Even now, with so much known about AIDS, some individuals hold to the misconception that AIDS is transmitted through the air or contact with skin (Hatfield & Dunkel, 1988). In many instances, misinformed persons, although well intentioned, may overreact and suggest that others beware of co-workers suspected of belonging to a high-risk group (Dilley, Batki & Shelp, 1987). Not only do employees who work with HIV-infected persons fear that they will contract the disease, but also they have irrational fears that they or their clothes are contaminated and that they will bring the disease to their families and friends (Hatfield & Dunkel, 1988). Such fears are apparent as these workers wear more protective clothing than necessary.

Homophobia and Fear of Other Lifestyle Behaviors

Because most AIDS victims have been homosexual or bisexual men or IV drug users, AIDS engenders in many people strong fears regarding sexuality and drug use. These fears may be a result of our own unresolved feelings about homosexuality or other lifestyle behaviors (Lewis, 1988). Historically, society views homosexuals, drug users, and prostitutes with suspicion and stigmatizes persons in these groups. Fear may produce a tendency to blame these victims for the tragedy of AIDS (Dilley, Batki & Shelp, 1987). Never before have we had so pressing a need to confront the issues of sexuality and drugs in relation to our coworkers. Few such emotional issues are to be found in the workplace.

Overidentification

Additional reactions such as overidentification and anger result when a coworker is found to have AIDS. Developmentally, most AIDS patients as young adults are beginning to establish identities, careers, and intimate relationships. At this time in their lives, they are not yet financially secure, nor do they have strong social support (Christ & Wiener, 1985). Coworkers who are also in this stage of life identify with the person with AIDS. Often coworkers experience "symptoms" and think that they too have developed AIDS. Anxiety, frustration, bodily concern, and anger can be manifested. In some situations, coworkers may become involved to compensate for their own feelings and may invest unrealistic amounts of time and energy in assisting the individual with AIDS. In other situations, coworkers may distance themselves from the worker with AIDS in order to reduce the overidentification and resulting feelings of guilt.

Fear of Death and Dying

Seeing a coworker battling a terminal disease is traumatic. AIDS results in good days and bad days, fatigue, and hospitalizations. The progressive development of AIDS with low reserves physically and emotionally is characteristic of the disease (Dilley, Batki & Shelp, 1987). Some employees may be unable to face the changes in physical appearance and the physical deterioration of a coworker. Some individuals may be fearful of the dying person and think that somehow death may be contagious. Unresolved feelings about one's own mortality may be intensified as a result of working alongside someone with AIDS. Psychological conflicts may be generated and lead to difficulty in relating to the individual with AIDS. These difficulties are apparent in managers as well as line workers. For example, in dealing with the issue of death and dying, a manager may be more comfortable in trying to encourage an employee with AIDS to go on disability or resign, when in actuality the employee may have years of productive service left.

CURRENT KNOWLEDGE AND ATTITUDES REGARDING AIDS

Considering the need for a proactive workplace response to AIDS, managers and occupational health professionals can benefit from recent surveys of public knowledge and attitudes regarding AIDS. These data can be helpful in planning educational and psychological approaches to AIDS in the workplace.

From August to December 1987, the National Health Interview Survey, routinely conducted by the U.S. Bureau of the Census to obtain health information, included AIDS knowledge and attitudes questions. The AIDS questions developed by working groups from the National Center for Health Statistics; the Centers for Disease Control, the National Institutes of Health; the Alcohol, Drug Abuse and Mental Health Administration, and the Health Resources and Services Administration were designed to collect baseline information on public knowledge and attitudes regarding the transmission and prevention of AIDS. Data will also be collected at future intervals to determine changes in knowledge and attitudes in the American population.

The National Health Interview Survey questionnaire included items on self-assessment of knowledge about AIDS, sources of information about AIDS, knowledge about AIDS and AIDS-related risk factors, modes of transmission, and blood tests for the AIDS virus; plans to take such a test, recent experience with blood donation, self-assessment of chances of getting AIDS, personal knowledge of people with AIDS or the AIDS virus, and finally, willingness to take part in a proposed national seroprevelance study.

The National Health Interview Survey is a continuous, cross-sectional household interview survey. A probability sample of the civilian noninstitutionalized population was selected and 2,303 (81 percent) of the sample completed interviews. A single randomly chosen adult (over age 18) in each selected household was interviewed.

Provisional results from the survey indicated that virtually everyone (more than 99 percent) has heard of AIDS. Almost three-fourths of adults (74 percent) last saw, heard, or read something about AIDS within three days of the NHIS interview. Twenty percent of adults 18 years of age and over feel that they know a lot about AIDS (compared to most people); 40 percent feel they know some; 30 percent feel they know a little; and 10 percent feel they know nothing about AIDS. Adults 50 years and over are more likely than younger adults to state that they know nothing about AIDS and less likely to think that they know a lot. Black respondents (17 percent) are almost twice as likely as white respondents (9 percent) to state that they know nothing about AIDS.

The majority of respondents are certain that AIDS leads to death (89 percent) and that no cure for AIDS exists at present (83 percent). Three-fourths of adults think that anyone with the AIDS virus definitely can transmit it to other individuals through sexual intercourse; another 18 percent think that the statement is probably true. About two-thirds of the adults in the United States definitely think that AIDS can cripple the body's natural protection against disease and that a pregnant woman can transmit AIDS to her baby.

Respondents are less certain about the causes of AIDS and about the relationship between the AIDS virus and the disease

AIDS: 44 percent of adults definitely believe that a virus causes AIDS, and 31 percent think that this is probably true; 50 percent are certain that a person can be infected with the AIDS virus and not have the disease AIDS, and 27 percent think that this is probably true. Adults are less informed about the specific ways that AIDS can affect its victims than about its causes; for example, 24 percent are certain that the AIDS virus can damage the brain. For the most part, the lowest levels of general knowledge are found among adults 50 years of age and over, consistent with their own self-assessment as a group that they know relatively little about the disease.

Most Americans are aware of the ways in which the AIDS virus is likely to be transmitted. More than 9 out of 10 adults say that a person is very likely to get AIDS from having sex with a person who has AIDS (92 percent) or by sharing needles for drug use with someone who has AIDS (91 percent). Conversely, the level of misinformation about modes of transmission, particularly from casual contact, is very high. For example, donating blood is considered a likely mode of transmission by 25 percent; working near someone with AIDS by 21 percent; sharing eating utensils with someone who has AIDS by 47 percent; using public toilets by 31 percent; and being bitten by mosquitoes or other insects by 38 percent.

Black respondents are significantly more likely than white respondents to perceive a threat of AIDS virus infection from receiving a blood transfusion, donating blood, using public toilets, or various other types of casual contact with persons who have AIDS. Few differences exist by age, sex, and marital status in knowledge or misinformation about the transmission of AIDS.

A number of questions were asked about blood tests for the AIDS virus. Overall, 70 percent of adults have heard of the blood test. Persons 30 to 49 years of age are most likely (79 percent) and persons 50 years of age and older are least likely (57 percent) to have heard of the test. Although respondents are widely aware that a blood test for the AIDS virus is available, they appear to have some misunderstanding about the purpose of the test. Forty-one percent of adults (58 percent of those who have heard of the test) erroneously believe that the blood test results tell whether a person has AIDS.

Seven percent of respondents report having had their blood tested for the AIDS virus, including 2 percent who voluntarily said that they were tested because of a blood donation or transfusion. (However, about 12 percent report having given blood since January 1985, the approximate date when routine testing of donated blood began.) These provisional data indicate that adults under age 30 are about four times as likely to have had the AIDS blood test as persons 50 years of age and over. In addition, 11 percent of all adults have thought about having the AIDS test, and 4 percent say that they plan to be tested in the next 12 months. Twelve percent of Americans age 18 years and over say they know someone who has had the AIDS blood test.

Most adults believe that they (and the people that they know) are at little or no risk of AIDS virus infection. Nine in 10 feel that they have no chance (60 percent) or a low chance (30 percent) of getting AIDS themselves. Six in 10 say that the chance of someone they know getting AIDS is low (34 percent) or nonexistent (26 percent). Six percent of adults report personally knowing someone with the AIDS virus.

Almost 9 of 10 Americans realize that both celibacy and restricting sexual activity to a monogamous relationship with a person who does not have the AIDS virus are very effective ways to avoid infection with the AIDS virus. One-third (34 percent) think that using condoms is a very effective way to avoid the virus, and an additional 48 percent consider this method somewhat effective. Slightly more than half of the adults in the United States (56 percent) think that using a diaphragm is not an effective way to avoid infection with the AIDS virus. An almost equal proportion (54 percent) feel that using spermicides is ineffective in AIDS prevention.

Two-thirds of adults (67 percent) have discussed AIDS with friends or relatives. Persons age 50 and over are the least likely to have done so. Of adults with children between the ages of 10 and 17, 60 percent report having talked with their children about AIDS (12 percent of all adults), and just over one-third of those with children in this age range report that their children have received instruction about AIDS at school.

In addition, 21 percent of the respondents thought that getting AIDS from working near someone with AIDS was very likely or somewhat likely. Forty-one percent thought that getting AIDS from being coughed or sneezed on by someone with AIDS was very likely or somewhat likely. Twelve percent thought getting AIDS from shaking hands or touching someone with AIDS very likely or somewhat likely.

KNOWLEDGE AND ATTITUDES TOWARD WORKERS WITH AIDS

Recently published reports provide data on the attitudes and behavioral intentions of individuals toward an HIV-positive coworker. Herold (1988) conducted a national probability survey of 2,000 workers over age 18 and found that large portions of the sample had concerns about working with persons who have AIDS. Two-thirds of the sample (66 percent) would be concerned about sharing bathroom facilities, and 40 percent were fearful about eating in the same cafeteria. Over one-third (37 percent) responded that they would be unwilling to share work tools and equipment with a coworker who has AIDS. Results indicate that fear and concern about coworkers with AIDS are prevalent at this time and could potentially disrupt workplace operations.

In another study, Hansen, Booth, Fawal, and Langner (1988) surveyed 198 subjects to ascertain their attitudes toward coworkers with AIDS. The sample included 53 nurses and laboratory technologists at a private hospital, 73 white-collar workers and computer programmers at an urban university, and 68 blue-collar building service workers at the same university. Items on the survey instrument measured attitudes toward AIDS and subjects' intended actions when in contact with an HIV-positive coworker.

The respondents ranged in age from 20 to 65 years. Most of the subjects were female (70 percent) and married (53 percent). Eighteen percent of the subjects indicated that they handled blood or body fluids of clients. In contrast, only two respondents (1 percent) indicated having a coworker who had tested positive for the AIDS virus. Most subjects (61 percent) did not know if they had a coworker who tested positive for the AIDS virus.

Subjects indicated positive behavioral intentions toward a coworker who was HIV positive in the following areas: continuing casual conversation (90 percent), carpooling (67 percent), sharing an office (72 percent), shaking hands (67 percent), eating in the same cafeteria (79 percent), and eating at the same table (68 percent). Blue-collar workers measured 3 to 4 percentage points lower on the items than the health-care and white-collar workers.

Responses to other items indicated either a lack of knowledge or disregard of what experts state are the modes of AIDS transmission. The majority of respondents (60 percent) would not share a unisex bathroom with a coworker who had tested positive for the AIDS virus. Eighty-one percent of the subjects would not eat food prepared by the coworker who had tested positive for the AIDS virus. One explanation may be fear that food preparers could cut themselves and spill blood into the food. Of further interest is that 61 percent of the respondents would not invite the coworker home for dinner. The responses of the blue-collar workers were more negative on these items than either the health-care workers or white-collar workers.

When asked what action they would take if they learned that a coworker had been diagnosed with AIDS, 55 percent would continue as if nothing had changed, 35 percent would avoid contact as much as possible, and two subjects would try to get the employee terminated. A number of subjects commented they would continue working but added some stipulations. Most related to taking precautions in their contact with the coworker. Three respondents commented that they would try to be supportive and help the coworker cope. Another subject would try not to say the wrong thing but would change the working conditions if they were physically close.

Two respondents' comments reflected some of the fear of AIDS. "I would make a greater effort to talk to the person, and to have minor contact such as a pat on the back. On the other hand, I would be avoiding contact with any body fluids — this includes moisture droplets from a sneeze. I know the experts say just blood and semen, but I don't trust that." Another subject stated, "Continue working with the coworker provided a mutual understanding is reached concerning some sense of fear I would have about contracting the disease through daily contact." This subject's lack of understanding about transmission is similar to that of other subjects who would avoid touching objects used in common. Another subject commented, "The disease is a different story than testing positive for an antibody. I would stay clear if the person had the disease."

In contrast to findings in the literature, two-thirds of the subjects (65 percent) would not care how the coworker contracted the AIDS virus. Whether the lack of concern is due to an absence of negative feelings toward homosexuals or to the question not accurately measuring the researchers' intent is not clear. Most respondents (72 percent) indicated they were somewhat knowledgeable about AIDS, 10 percent indicated they were not knowledgeable, and 18 percent believed they were very knowledgeable.

The differences between the groups with regard to their knowledge level was very interesting. Forty percent of the health-care workers and 13 percent of the blue-collar non-health-care workers rated themselves very knowledgeable about AIDS. In contrast, only 8 percent of the white-collar non-health-care workers believed they were very knowledgeable about AIDS. However, almost one-fourth of the blue-collar non-health-care workers indicated that they were not knowledgeable, compared to 2 percent of the health-care workers and 5 percent of the white-collar non-health-care workers.

The sources of information about AIDS varied considerably. Sixty-nine percent of the blue-collar non-health-care workers obtained all of their information about AIDS from the media. Only five of those employees had ever attended an in-service on AIDS. Additionally, only six of the white-collar non-health-care workers had attended an AIDS in-service program. In contrast, 33 of the 52 health-care workers had obtained knowledge about AIDS from an in-service program. One-quarter of the respondents indicated that word of mouth was a source of knowledge.

Workers' beliefs about mandatory AIDS testing by employers also showed variations. More of the computer programmers (46 percent) favored mandatory testing than did the building service personnel (29 percent) or nurses and laboratory technologists (29 percent). Of the subjects who felt mandatory testing was appropriate, 65 percent indicated that all employees should be tested. Nine subjects felt health-care professionals should be tested and six subjects believed food-handlers should be tested. One subject stated that testing should not be mandatory, but that free testing should be available. Another subject commented that testing should definitely not be mandatory because the "test is not all inclusive and can be misleading—sets people up to be discriminated against."

A statistical test, the Kruskall-Wallis one-way ANOVA, revealed a significant difference between the blue-collar, white-collar, and health-care workers. The health-care workers had more positive behavioral intentions than the non-health-care workers. The behavioral intentions of the white-collar workers were more positive than the blue-collar workers.

RECOMMENDATIONS

A synthesis of the literature and research on workers' fears and attitudes provides a number of recommendations for managers and occupational health professionals trying to achieve more positive reactions to AIDS in the workplace:

1. Alert managers, supervisors, and other employees that the company will focus on providing education and support to assist the employees in dealing with their emotional reactions.

2. Help employees express their fears in positive ways such as through educational seminars and group counseling.
3. Conduct AIDS educational programs on a regular basis to provide updates and a forum for discussion.
4. Help employees express acceptance, hope, and support to coworkers with AIDS.
5. Encourage employees to seek confidential support through an employee assistance program.
6. Encourage employee participation on task forces to set AIDS policies in the workplace.
7. Offer educational programs and counseling for the families of employees who are concerned about working with someone with AIDS.
8. Correct inaccuracies and rumors about AIDS in the company.

SUMMARY

If any single theme runs through this chapter, it is that emotional reactions to an epidemic such as AIDS are natural and to be expected. Fear and avoidance of coworkers who are HIV positive will no doubt be demonstrated in the workplace. Time spent developing policy, education, and counseling strategies will be more than regained when a company has its first case of AIDS.

REFERENCES

Business Leadership Task Force (1986) *AIDS in the Workplace Manual.* (Available from the San Francisco AIDS Foundation, 333 Valencia Street, Fourth Floor, San Francisco, California 94103).

Christ, G., & L. Wiener (1985) Psychosocial issues in AIDS. In V. DeVita, S. Hellman & S. Rosenberg, eds., *AIDS: Etiology, Diagnosis, Treatment and Prevention,* pp. 275-297. Philadelphia: J. B. Lippincott.

Dilley, J., S. Batki & E. Shelp (1987) Psychiatric and ethical issues in the care of patients with AIDS. In M. Helquist, ed., *Working with AIDS,* pp. 247-255. San Francisco: AIDS Health Project.

Hansen, B., W. Booth, H. Fawal & R. Langner (1988) Workers with AIDS: Attitudes of fellow employees. *American Association of Occupational Health Nurses Journal* 36:279-283.

Hatfield, S., & J. Dunkel (1988) Understanding and working with the emotional reactions of staff. In A. Lewis, ed., *Nursing Care of the Person with AIDS,* pp. 259-275. Rockville, Maryland: Aspen Publishers, Inc.

Herold, D. M. (1988) Employees' Reactions to AIDS in the Workplace. Atlanta: Georgia Institute of Technology.

Lewis, A. (1988) Dealing with issues of sexuality. In A. Lewis, ed., *Nursing Care of the Person with AIDS/ARC,* pp. 283-286. Rockville, Maryland: Aspen Publishers, Inc.

National Center for Health Statistics, D. Dawson, M. Cynamon & J. Fitti (1987) AIDS knowledge and attitudes, provisional data from the National Health Interview Survey: United States, August 1987. *Advance Data from Vital and Health Statistics* (No. 146, DHHS Publication No. 88-1250). Hyattsville, Maryland: United States Public Health Service.

Quinn, T. (1987) The acquired immune deficiency syndrome (AIDS). Presented at the Association for Practitioners in Infection Control Annual Educational Conference, Miami, Florida.

Turner, J., D. Gauthier, K. Ellison & D. Griener (1988) Nursing and AIDS: Knowledge and attitudes. *American Association of Occupational Health Nurses Journal* 36:274-277.

8.

THE HIV-INFECTED EMPLOYEE

People who are informed that they are antibody positive for the human immunodeficiency virus (HIV) or HIV infected experience a variety of psychological, social, and even physical reactions over varying time periods. Reactions may depend on how well the individual understands the difference between being presumably infected with the HIV virus versus experiencing the specific signs and symptoms associated with AIDS-related conditions. Skilled pre- and post-test counseling should be conducted in conjunction with all AIDS testing so that the individual being tested is informed of what the test does and does not mean. As was discussed in chapter 1, any given individual who is antibody positive may or may not develop

---

Major portions of this chapter were reproduced from the July 1988 *AAOHN Journal* special issue on AIDS with permission of the *American Association of Occupational Health Nurses' Journal* and Slack Publishing Company. The original article, "Nurse management of the HIV-infected employee," was written by Karen D. Newman, Ann Sirles, and Kenny M. Williamson.

disease in the months or years ahead. Although the current belief is that the majority of HIV-infected individuals will experience disease symptoms at some time in the future, possibly new drugs will become available that will either keep the viral particles inactivated and therefore retard or stop disease development, or even act to kill the HIV virus and render the individual noninfectious. Looking for a drug or drugs that will "cure" the HIV-infected individual is considered fantasy by some and merely a race against time by others. In either case, the uncertainty of treatment for the disease contributes to HIV-infected individuals' sense of profound helplessness.

Regardless of how HIV infection occurs, the universal feelings of anger, fear, some degree of bereavement, and a sense of social stigma are experienced by affected individuals and their families. The individual and/or family may fear discovery by other members of the community, church, school, or workplace. Further, because most HIV-infected individuals are relatively young, they are generally unprepared for what may well be a terminal illness and can be expected to experience feelings of grief and anger regardless of how well or how ill they are when notified of their antibody status.

MAJOR TREATMENT STRATEGIES

Although AIDS has been a universally fatal disease to date, being told that one is antibody or HIV positive is not equivalent to being diagnosed with AIDS. Because many HIV-positive people are experiencing relatively good health when they are initially identified, both contemporary and evolving medical and health-management strategies might greatly slow or conceivably even halt progression of the disease process. The two goals of health management of HIV-infected people are essentially to prolong life and decrease the frequency and severity of infections and rare cancers associated with autoimmune states.

Drug Treatment

The first goal of health management involves preventing further damage to the immune system, and the second goal is to prevent or to diagnose infections at very early stages of development (Ziegler, 1987). Drugs can be used to stop the multiplication of the HIV virus, to boost the immune system, and to treat associated opportunistic infections. That is, drugs can be used if their toxic side effects can be tolerated so that the therapeutic benefit outweighs side effects. The bottom line is that for the HIV-infected individual, survival may be contingent upon how well these two treatment objectives can be managed both by the patient and by the health-care provider.

The primary drug intervention at this time is the use of azidothymidine (AZT), an antiviral agent that inhibits replication of the HIV virus. It is prescribed for a two-year course of therapy and requires that the individual take 200 mg of the medication every 4 hours around the clock. Red blood cell and white blood cell counts are monitored monthly to ascertain the effects of the drug on the body. This medication costs $700 to 800 per month. Other medications such as immune stimulants and drugs to treat specific opportunistic infections may also be prescribed.

The employer needs to understand that HIV-infected people who are taking various drugs require frequent systematic appraisals of the drug's effect on the body. Sometimes the medications needed must be administered by a health professional either at home or in a health-care facility.

Maintenance of a Healthy Immune System

Keeping the immune system healthy, or at least lessening further insult to the immune system, is one way in which infections associated with AIDS-related diseases can be potentially delayed or avoided. Keeping the immune system healthy requires good general health-promotion techniques and involves many aspects of daily living. For example, a key requisite for a healthy immune system is adequate nutrition and rest. Yet, one of the early and persistent problems experienced by people with AIDS-related diseases is chronic fatigue and weight loss due to a combination of physiologic and emotional factors. Although the severity of symptoms varies with each individual, in general, people with HIV-related disease require more rest and a higher protein and overall calorie intake to avoid depressing an already compromised immune system.

Aside from adequate nutrition and rest, HIV-infected individuals must reduce those factors in their lives that are known to disrupt immune functioning. Therefore, they usually require specific counseling regarding stress management, safer sex practices, and absolute avoidance of alcohol and non-prescribed drugs.

Clearly, removing all stressors from a person's life is neither possible nor desirable. The point is that when the HIV-infected individual experiences unmanageable degrees of stress, the immune function may be further compromised. For these reasons, usually the individual must learn effective measures for dealing with perceived stressors, including psychiatric or mental health counseling, if needed, and the use of community-based support groups. Incorporating an appropriate degree of exercise into the health regimen is also important.

Little consensus exists among experts as to why AIDS-related diseases occur early in some HIV-infected persons and later or conceivably not at all in others. However, not only is reexposure to the virus believed to increase chances of becoming initially infected, but reexposure to the virus is also believed to prompt activation of HIV in the infected individual and result subsequently in clinical manifestations of the disease. For this reason, HIV-infected individuals must be taught to avoid sex or drug behavior that might result in reexposure to HIV. Avoidance of drug behaviors includes avoiding all forms of alcohol, including beer, wine, and hard liquor. Not only does alcohol intake tend to suppress immune functioning but also it alters judgment in that inebriated persons are more apt to engage in risky sexual practices. The same is true of other types of drugs like marijuana and cocaine. So the HIV-infected individual must be taught how to prevent injury and insult to the immune system.

Treatment for HIV Infections

The second treatment or management strategy revolves around either prophylactic treatment or early diagnosis and treatment of the various infections known to occur in HIV-infected people. Toward this end, HIV-infected individuals, *regardless of their subjective or objective health status, should be examined by a professional health-care provider at least every six months.* The goal of these evaluations is to assess the relative integrity of the immune system and to start infected individuals on drugs known to prevent or lessen the occurrence of specific AIDS-related diseases as early as is clinically indicated. Additionally, infected individuals should be carefully counseled about systematic methods of monitoring their bodily functions such as temperature, weight, and degree of fatigue. The philosophy behind this strategy is that the individual will be able to detect early changes or symptoms and seek timely health-care intervention.

STAGES OF HIV INFECTION

Whether the HIV-infected employee uses accrued sick time or continues to work at all depends upon a combination of factors that include company policy, employer attitude, personal need, and stage of disease. However, the stage of disease being experienced will by and large determine the individual's physical and emotional ability to function productively in the work setting. In rare instances, the HIV-infected employee will need assistance with decision making relative to continuing in the work setting.

As discussed in chapter 1, the first stage in AIDS-related disorders is asymptomatic HIV infection. The affected individual may feel quite well and therefore be unaware of the infection. Even careful physical examination may not reveal any AIDS-associated phenomena like swollen lymph glands or weight loss. A small percentage of HIV-infected individuals may not progress beyond this stage, especially if they practice good overall health habits and avoid reinfection.

These individuals are physically capable of working in virtually any work setting so long as they can simultaneously control exposure to immunosuppressive agents such as ionizing radiation. Further, they pose no risk of infection to coworkers, assuming no sexual or direct blood contact, and assuming that the employee in question is able to control bodily functions. Sharing restroom and kitchen or dining facilities with coworkers poses no hazard because AIDS is not transmitted by toilet seats or food any more than gonorrhea or syphilis is.

Regardless of their lack of physical signs and symptoms, HIV-infected individuals should be evaluated every six months by a health-care professional who is informed about their antibody status. Also, because antibody-positive individuals are presumed HIV infected and capable of transmitting the virus, they should be counseled carefully about how to contain their infection. For example, they should practice scrupulous personal hygiene, practice sexual abstinence or safer sex, should not donate blood or body organs, and should make provisions for preventing pregnancy.

Once asymptomatic HIV-infected persons begin to manifest various AIDS-related signs and symptoms, they can be placed into the early, middle, or late stages of the disease. The early or acute phase is marked by one or more bouts of acute infection between long periods of time when the person feels relatively well. During the middle or chronic phase, the infections and/or cancer become chronically debilitating, and in the end stage the person nears death and is actively dying (Moed & Kline, 1988).

During the second stage of health deterioration associated with AIDS-related disease, generalized symptoms of fatigue, weight loss, swollen lymph nodes, and night sweats may continue or be experienced intermittently, but some specific AIDS-related condition such as pneumonia or rare cancer like Kaposi's sarcoma frequently necessitates hospitalization for intensive treatment. For example, the worker may suffer intermittently from diarrhea so severe that working on a regular basis becomes impossible. The worker may also experience various neurological manifestations such as seizures, forgetfulness, loss of concentration, confusion, and marked impairment of recent memory. Although these kinds of symptoms most often occur later in the disease process, they can occur earlier. In some instances, the quality and quantity of work diminish noticeably. Therefore, AIDS-related policies must be flexible enough to support the HIV-infected employee who is performing well versus the one who is literally unable to function. In the latter case, the most obvious policy is to treat the HIV-infected employee like any other employee who is too ill to work.

Thus, in the second stage of disease, the employee may need to take medical leave from work for intensive home or hospital treatment. The individual may begin to wonder whether he or she will be able to continue to work. As often happens if the employee has not yet informed the worksite about the illness, the health-care insurer may be the one who notifies the employer that a particular employee has filed for compensation for an AIDS-related disease.

Acute episodes of infection may be followed by chronic phases in which the employee may not be bedridden but will most likely be unable to work. At this point, the individual may begin having difficulty in the activities of daily living, that is, food preparation and maintenance of living quarters. He or she may also be experiencing increasing and sometimes overwhelming fatigue that necessitates 12 or more hours of rest at a time. The individuals may also be experiencing increased outlay of money for prescriptions and over-the-counter medications to manage increasingly severe symptoms. Also, during this and all stages of illness to come, the individual and his or her family or significant others may be obsessed with locating treatment or even experimental programs. They have the common, if overly optimistic, feeling that the right combination of medications or nutrition or lifestyle alteration might "beat the disease."

If and when the individual is able to return to work, the employer should be aware that specific job functions may have to be changed or modified to less stressful or less physically demanding duties. At the very least, the work schedule must be flexible enough to allow the worker to keep the rather frequent evaluation and treatment appointments necessary to monitor and manage the disease process. As discussed in chapter 3, the HIV-infected employee should not be denied company benefits for health insurance, sick leave, and disability.

During the chronic stage, the individual usually becomes physically unable to work. Again, many years may separate the stages, and with drug therapy improving with time, an affected individual might live many years or perhaps never progress to the chronic and terminal stages of disease. In the late chronic stage and beginning terminal stages, the previously mentioned symptoms become unmanageable and seldom abate. Repeated infection or invasive cancer may cause profound physical changes such as loss of teeth, loss of muscle mass, and debilitation to the point that the individual is largely either homebound or even completely bedridden.

Progressing with grief reaction, fear of death, and occasional dementia brought about by the virus invading the brain, individuals may vacillate between depression, rage, dementia, euphoria, and points when they seem to fail to recognize significant people in their lives. Almost all require some form of attendant care and/or skilled home nursing. Health care costs, which may be devastating, are discussed in Chapter 2.

At some point, the now physically and emotionally ravaged individual begins what has been called "active dying" (Moed & Kline, 1988). Total and continuous care is required whether in the home with the help of hospice personnel or final hospitalization. Even death does not come predictably or easily.

ROLE OF THE OCCUPATIONAL HEALTH PROFESSIONAL

Emotional and Physical Support

Because AIDS-related conditions vary in clinical presentation and severity, the company occupational health physician or nurse may be called upon to manage a wide variety of associated problems and concerns among the work force. For example, employees may be concerned about being HIV infected, in which case information should be provided to employees about community resources for anonymous or confidential HIV-antibody testing. Additionally, it is likely that there will be numerous opportunities to answer AIDS-related questions as employees become more knowledgeable about how the disease is transmitted. As the number of people with AIDS-related illnesses grows, the occupational health professional will be called upon to care for affected workers in varying stages of wellness/illness.

To be maximally therapeutic, the two health-management strategies involving maintenance of a healthy immune system and early diagnosis and treatment of AIDS-related diseases must be understood. All strategies related to personal and group risk assessment (see chapter 11) as well as means for preventing transmission of HIV in a seemingly endless variety of situations must be addressed. Finally, as a first-line resource, the occupational health professional must be able to deal effectively with the psychosocial needs precipitated by HIV-related conditions and must provide emotional care for the HIV-infected person who is still relatively well. The worker who suffers from AIDS-related illnesses must be provided the emotional and psychosocial assistance needed to deal with a highly stigmatized terminal disease.

In counseling the known HIV-infected worker, the individual's fear of future illness as well as concerns regarding the reactions of family, friends, and coworkers should be recognized. Initially, an HIV-infected worker often expresses fear

and guilt over having possibly exposed family members and/or
sexual partners to the virus. At this time, education must be
provided regarding methods of transmission of the virus, stressing that HIV infection is not spread by casual contact. Additionally, workers may ask for assistance in teaching family
members about HIV infection. Sexual partners of infected
workers may need information as to HIV test sites in the community, and both workers and their sexual partners will need
information on "safer sex" practices to lower the chances of
HIV transmission.

As the worker overcomes the initial shock from the diagnosis of HIV infection, concern over possible illness grows. The
infected worker requires emotional support and assurance that
one episode of influenza, for example, is not indicative of
clinical AIDS. Stress management techniques may be geared to
alleviate some unnecessary fears.

For the worker diagnosed with an AIDS-related illness, the
psychosocial issues become even more complex. Although
most individuals experience anxiety and depression, physical
effects of anxiety may present in the form of overt tension,
tachycardia, agitation, anorexia, and panic attacks.

Employees with AIDS may also exhibit low self-esteem secondary to their depressed state. They are distressed and preoccupied with their own imminent illness and death. Symptoms
of depression such as a feeling of hopelessness or overt with-
drawal and social isolation are not uncommon. The worker
becomes angry at both the disease and the discrimination that
often accompanies the disease.

According to one author, AIDS can be described as "a series
of losses...health, friends, loved ones, home, economic independence, and the ability to carry out day-to-day tasks"
(Feinblum, 1986, p. 255). Because of the associated social
stigma, people with AIDS suffer greater loss in significant
relationships compared to people with other terminal illnesses.
These workers may feel a need to conceal their diagnosis for
fear of job loss, eviction by landlords, and public persecution.

The family, friends, lovers, and children of the worker are affected by the psychological repercussions of AIDS-related disease. Fears of relatives and friends may manifest in the form of anger, unrealistic guilt, and loss of emotional control. A relative diagnosed with AIDS may even be abandoned. Therefore, caring for workers with HIV-related disease and their families or significant others involves health promotion, client advocacy, and anticipatory guidance.

The challenge associated with HIV-related illness is at least twofold. The occupational health professional must deal not only with what can be a largely unfamiliar disease that is associated with fear, dread, death, and even hatred but also cope with personal fears about the disease while caring for employees. Added stressors in the workplace may result from displaced anger and hostility exhibited by people who are unnecessarily afraid of an infected coworker. Adequate preplanning and employee counseling and education may alleviate some of these difficulties.

Education and counseling for HIV-infected employees should be similar to points that should be known by the public at large and achieve the following four objectives:

- Present factual, current information on HIV infection and other HIV-related diseases such as ARC and AIDS and how they differ.
- Identify risk factors and explain how HIV infection is transmitted so as to allay fears about acquisition of HIV infection through the casual contact that would occur in the worksite.
- Discuss prevention of HIV infection and promotion of health habits to achieve optimum health.
- Provide information about community resources for anonymous or confidential HIV-antibody testing, the existence of community-based support groups, and local and national AIDS hotlines where questions can be answered by experts at virtually any time of day.

Casefinding

During the course of routine periodic physical examinations, health professionals may encounter the worker who has AIDS-related symptomatology (see chapter 1). Most of the initial signs and symptoms of such diseases are nonspecific but persistent and chronic. The most common signs and symptoms of AIDS-related diseases that may be discovered during a routine physical examination include diffuse lymphadenopathy, persistent diarrhea, weight loss and candidiasis. Additionally, the hairy leukoplakia frequently seen in AIDS-related disease states is so unusual that its presence in healthy adults should arouse strong suspicion of HIV exposure. Likewise, employees with severe herpes zoster (shingles) should receive a thorough history and physical examination.

Where workers are to be referred for further health care or evaluation depends on the resources within the community, company insurance parameters, and the worker's preference. Initially, however, the worker's rights to privacy must be protected, and appropriate emotional support must be provided. The American Association of Occupational Health Nurses has published *Guidelines for Confidentiality of Health Information,* which defines the levels of confidentiality, establishes protocols for access to health records, states the circumstances of disclosure of health information, and identifies a system to ensure the security of health records (AAOHN, 1988). In essence, the AAOHN guidelines identify three levels of confidentiality. Level III, personal health information, includes such areas as treatments for AIDS-related diseases as well as family health counseling related to HIV infection. The only situations under which this information may be released are:

- Life-threatening emergencies
- Employee-authorized release to insurance companies, personal physicians, and the like
- Worker's compensation claims
- Compliance with government regulations

Thus the occupational health nurse or physician, as primary provider of health care in the workplace, must be prepared to manage effectively the broad clinical spectrum of HIV infection in workers. This preparation, however, requires much more than an ability to provide physical care. Social and emotional support for workers who are HIV infected and/or those who have AIDS-related disorders provide a direct challenge to occupational health professionals. As the magnitude of the AIDS phenomenon increases, the company and the occupational health unit must develop confidential, caring policies and procedures in line with the overall workplace policy to assist HIV-infected workers in maintaining physical and psychosocial well-being as long as possible.

SUMMARY

Managing the HIV-infected employee from an employer standpoint depends in part on the previous employer-employee relationship, the nature of individual workplace policy, and the extent of physical and emotional debilitation experienced in conjunction with progressive disease. Whether AIDS will continue to be considered a universally fatal disease and how many HIV-infected individuals actually progress to AIDS are highly contingent upon development of and access to effective treatments, including a growing arsenal of drugs. The day may well come when HIV infection is placed on a parallel with chronic tuberculosis or hepatitis in that the individual may continue to work throughout the life span so long as treatment regimes are followed. Until then, every employer must treat each HIV-infected individual with the dignity and opportunity afforded to any worker whose health may be compromised.

REFERENCES

American Association of Occupational Health Nurses (1988) Guidelines for confidentiality of health information.

American Association of Occupational Health Nurses' Journal 36(1):6–7.

Feinblum, S. (1986) Pinning down the psychosocial dimensions of AIDS. *Nursing and Health Care* 7(5):255–257.

Moed, A., & A.Kline (1988) Discharge planning. In A. Lewis, ed., *Nursing Care of the Person with AIDS/ARC*, pp. 205–210. Rockville, Maryland: Aspen Corporation.

Newman, K. D., A. Sirles & K. M. Williamson (1988) Nurse management of the HIV-infected employee. *American Association of Occupational Health Nurses' Journal* 36(7):258–261.

Ziegler, J. (1987) Treatment and prevention of AIDS. In B. C. Moffatt, J. Spiegel, S. Parrish & M. Helquist, eds., *AIDS: A Self-Care Manual*, pp. 107–116. Los Angeles: AIDS Project.

9.

PROTECTING WORKERS FROM HIV INFECTION

All employers in the United States have been charged by the Occupational Safety and Health Administration (OSHA) to provide employees with safe and healthful working conditions (Department of Labor, 1987). Included in this responsibility is the duty to take specific actions to protect workers against bloodborne viruses such as the human immunodeficiency virus (HIV) and the virus that causes hepatitis B or HBV. Protecting workers requires an understanding of how bloodborne viruses are transmitted and then careful examination of OSHA

Some portions of this chapter were reproduced from the July 1988 *AAOHN Journal* special issue on AIDS with permission of the *American Association of Occupational Health Nurses Journal* and Slack Publishing Company. The original article, "Preventing HIV Transmission," was written by Joan Turner, Hala Fawal, Martha Long, and Margaret Rivers.

guidelines that delineate what may reasonably be expected of employers in this regard.

Once again, HIV is transmitted in three ways: from pregnant woman to fetus or newborn, by sexual contact, and by exposure to blood and other infectious body fluids. In this regard, the dangerous body fluids are blood, semen, and cerebrospinal fluid. Workplace exposure to other body fluids such as urine, feces, sweat, and tears are not associated with risk of HIV infection (CDC, 1988).

Because acquired immunodeficiency syndrome (AIDS) can be transmitted as a result of incidental or accidental exposure to infected blood or body tissues, workplace duties and expectations sometimes place the employee at varying risk for occupational exposure to HIV. Although the nation's 7 million health-care workers may be at highest risk for occupational exposure, any employee who comes in contact with infected blood or body fluids is at risk of infection. In late 1988, the Centers for Disease Control (CDC) reported a total of 16 health-care workers who had been HIV infected through their job activities in health-care settings. Each documented episode involved accidental needlestick injury or splashes of infected blood onto broken skin. Universal barrier precautions, as recommended by CDC (1987, 1988), when vigorously practiced will prevent such accidents. To date, no cases of HIV infections have been reported as occupationally induced in non-health-care workers, and the basic principles used with barrier precautions can be modified to cover literally any work setting.

OSHA GUIDELINES

When OSHA's guidelines relative to the prevention of exposure to HIV in the workplace appeared in the *Federal Register* (DOL, 1987), three categories of tasks were identified, ranging from Category I, those tasks that involve routine exposure to blood, body fluids, or tissues that may be potentially HIV infected, to Category III, those job tasks that involve no exposure to infected blood or body fluids (see Appendix D). Category II workers are those workers who do not have routine exposure to HIV-infected blood or tissues, but whose job functions may occasionally require the worker to come in contact with blood and other body fluids. Examples of Category II workers include police, firefighters, ambulance drivers, and first-aid-trained individuals who may be designated as "first responders" when a workplace injury occurs.

Workers included in Category I are defined as those who have job-related tasks that involve an inherent potential for mucous membrane or skin contact with human blood or tissues, or they are at risk of being splashed with infected body fluids. Only health-care workers, morticians, or those who work directly with human blood or blood products in health-care settings or laboratories qualify as Category I workers:

Dental assistants	Nursing assistants
Dental hygienists	Oral surgeons
Dentists	Paramedics
Laboratory workers	Phlebotomists
Medical assistants	Physician's assistants
Medical technologists	Physicians
Mortician assistants	Scrub (operating room)
Morticians	technicians
Nurses	Surgeons

Employer responsibility revolves around education and training on barrier precautions and making certain that required protective coverings are provided for each worker. Appropriate protective coverings include latex or vinyl gloves, gowns or plastic aprons, surgical masks and goggles (or a clear faceplate that protects both eyes and mouth), and one-way-valved face masks for administering mouth-to-mouth resuscitation.

Category II workers, according to OSHA, are those whose job tasks do *not* involve routine exposure to blood, body fluids, or tissues, but some aspects or conditions of employment may require the worker to perform Category I tasks. In other words, the normal job tasks do not routinely involve exposure to blood and body fluids, but occasional exposure may be required as a condition of employment. As mentioned previously, Category II subsumes a variety of workers such as those who might render first aid in emergency situations like firefighters and law enforcement personnel, and also relates to other workers such as sanitarians or even plumbers or maintenance personnel who may be required to clean or service environmental surfaces or equipment that is potentially contaminated with blood or body fluids. Overall employer responsibility to Category II workers is to identify, train, and provide ready access to protective equipment that can be used in emergency situations.

Category III workers are those whose usual job tasks involve no exposure to blood, body fluids, or tissues, and those who are not specifically charged with responsibilities that would place them at risk to those exposures. Although situations can be imagined or hypothesized under which anyone, anywhere, might encounter potential exposure to body fluids to some degree, the differentiation between Category II and Category III workers is essentially job expectations. For example, law enforcement personnel would be expected to render first aid as well as to apprehend and subdue others, and contact with blood is a possibility. In essence, employees who perform Category III duties are not called upon as a part of their employment to perform or assist in emergency medical care, or to be exposed in some other way. Handling of implements or utensils (as required for cooks or dishwashers), use of public or shared bathroom facilities or telephones, and personal contacts such as handshaking are all Category III tasks.

Examining the above three categories of tasks clarifies why many health-care workers are included in Category I and why employees such as police may well fall into Category II. However, the great majority of the work force, such as factory and office workers, falls within Category III. OSHA requirements for workers in the third category do not include specifications for protective strategies because this group is not considered to have an occupational risk of exposure to HIV as a part of their assigned job tasks. OSHA is expected to develop a formal standard for workplace exposure to bloodborne diseases in the near future.

UNIVERSAL BARRIER PRECAUTIONS

In order to prevent the spread of HIV infection, universal barrier precautions recommended by CDC (see Appendices F and G) must be adopted not only in hospitals but also in all job settings where Category I and/or II tasks are assigned to employees (CDC, 1987, 1988). Managers and occupational health personnel need to examine the risk of HIV infection in light of the nature of exposure in the work setting. For example, in worksites where the chance of emergency trauma is likely, whether or not the clinical or infectivity status of the employee is known, policies and mechanisms for implementing barrier precautions should be in place. The whole notion of barrier precautions is to provide a physical barrier that acts to prevent blood exposure to unprotected skin or mucous membranes (the mouth, nose, and eyes).

All workers should routinely use appropriate barrier precautions to prevent skin and mucous membrane exposure whenever contact with blood or other body fluids of any person is likely or can be anticipated. Gloves should be worn for touching blood and body fluids, mucous membranes, or nonintact skin, and for handling items or surfaces soiled with blood and/or body fluids. Disposable gloves are indicated to protect the skin when, for instance, stopping the bleeding of an accident victim. Disposable gloves should never be reused, but more rugged protective gloves, such as those that might be worn by housekeeping or maintenance personnel, can be cleaned and reused to protect skin.

To prevent exposure of the mucous membranes of the mouth, nose, and eyes, masks and protective eyewear or face shields should be worn during procedures likely to generate droplets of blood or other body fluids. For example, dentists and dental hygienists are at high risk of such spattered blood and are therefore urged to wear gloves and face shields. Additionally, gowns or aprons should be worn during procedures that are likely to generate splashes of blood or other body fluids (CDC, 1987).

Hands and other skin surfaces should be washed immediately and thoroughly if contaminated with blood or body fluids. Also, hands should be washed immediately after gloves are removed. The idea is to avoid leaving blood in contact with skin or mucous surfaces for a prolonged period of time, and washing vigorously with hand soap and water is all that is required to reduce risk of infection. For additional barrier precautions, especially relevant to health-care workers, see Appendices F and G.

All first-aid kits should include disposable gloves and other protective gear as might be indicated by the peculiarities of the work setting. Another important piece of equipment is the one-way-valved face mask that facilitates mouth-to-mouth resuscitation without extensive exposure to mucous membranes.

Hazardous Body Fluids

According to CDC, universal barrier precautions apply to human blood and other body fluids containing visible blood because occupational transmission of bloodborne diseases to health-care workers has been documented. Although not yet implicated in occupational transmission, the following body fluids are considered potentially infectious and universal precautions should be utilized when occupational exposure to them is likely:

- Semen and vaginal secretions
- Cerebrospinal fluid in the brain and spinal column
- Synovial fluid in and around joints such as knees
- Pleural fluid (found in the chest cavity)
- Peritoneal fluid (found in the abdominal cavity)

- Pericardial fluid (found in the walls of the heart)
- Amniotic fluid (bathes and protects the fetus)
- Any other body fluid mixed with visible blood

Saliva has not been implicated in HIV transmission, but oral secretions that are contaminated with blood pose a potential infection hazard. CDC guidelines (1988) specified that universal precautions do not apply to feces, nasal secretions, sputum (saliva), sweat, tears, urine, and vomitus *unless they contain visible blood,* because the risk of transmission of bloodborne viruses from these fluids and materials is extremely low or nonexistent.

ENVIRONMENTAL SANITATION

No environmental mode of HIV transmission has been documented, and current knowledge indicates that HIV is not transmitted by inanimate objects or surfaces that are not themselves heavily contaminated with live viral particles in blood spills. Extraordinary attempts to disinfect or sterilize environmental surfaces such as walls, floors, and other surfaces are not necessary. However, from a hygienic standpoint, cleaning and removal of soil should be done routinely (CDC, 1987).

Ordinary chemical germicides approved for use as hospital disinfectants or a 1:10 dilution of sodium hypochlorite (household bleach) may be used to decontaminate spills of blood and other body fluids when they occur. Gloves should be worn during the cleaning and decontaminating procedures (CDC, 1987).

Washable materials soiled with blood or body fluids should be placed in bags to prevent leakage. In general, clothing contaminated with blood should be detergent washed in water at least 71° C (160° F) for 25 minutes (CDC, 1987). In community settings or non-health-care facilities, soiled washables that are colorfast may be washed as usual with one cup of household chlorine bleach; noncolorfast materials can be washed with one-quarter cup of phenol solution.

PRECAUTIONS IN THE LABORATORY

All laboratory specimens should be treated as though infected. Any specimen knowingly taken from a person who is HIV infected should be clearly marked as a biohazard and transported in a leakproof container. Specimens leaking from their containers should ideally be discarded, but in those cases in which the specimen is not replaceable, the outside of the soiled container should be disinfected with a solution of 0.5 percent sodium hypochlorite spray and left standing for at least ten minutes before handling the specimen (Tierno, 1988).

Employers should also be aware that workers in laboratory settings should follow the book *Biosafety in Microbiological and Biomedical Laboratories ("Guidelines"),* which was originally developed by the CDC and the National Institutes of Health in consultation with experts from academic institutions, industry and government. Additionally, newer guidelines germane to laboratories were published by CDC in the April 1, 1988, issue of the *Morbidity and Mortality Weekly Report* (Vol. 37, No. s-4).

EMPLOYER RESPONSIBILITY

Essentially, OSHA has specified that employers have a responsibility to workers in the following areas, which will be elucidated in turn: training and education, engineering controls, work practices, personal protective equipment, medical services, and documentation or recordkeeping of potential hazards or actual incidents that may result in HIV infection (Department of Labor, 1987).

Training and Education

Initial and periodic training programs should be developed for all employees who perform Category I tasks (routine exposure to blood and body fluids) and/or Category II tasks (occasional exposure to blood and body fluids), and no worker should engage in any related task before receiving specific training aimed at the following points. Through employer-provided education and training, the employee will:

1. Understand how bloodborne viruses like HIV and HBV are transmitted from one person to another
2. Be able to recognize and differentiate between Category I and II tasks
3. Know the types of protective clothing and equipment appropriate for Category I and II tasks, and understand the basis for selection of specific protective clothing or equipment
4. Be familiar with appropriate actions to take and persons to contact if unplanned Category I tasks are encountered
5. Be familiar with and understand all the requirements for various work practices and protective equipment specified in written procedures that describe the task performed
6. Know where protective clothing and equipment is kept and how to use it properly, as well as be able to handle, decontaminate, and dispose of potentially contaminated clothing and equipment
7. Know and understand the limitations of protective clothing and equipment. For example, no amount of protective gear protects against accidental needle sticks
8. Know how to respond appropriately in the event of personal exposure to fluids or tissues, including the appropriate reporting procedures and medical monitoring recommended in such cases

Engineering Controls

Whenever possible, engineering controls should be utilized as the primary method to reduce worker exposure to real or potential hazards. For example, use of a laser scalpel is recommended to reduce the risks of cuts and scrapes that may result from handling conventional scalpel blades. Whenever any given job procedure results in a significant rate of injury to the worker, it should be carefully assessed and modified to reduce the chance of accidental injury.

Work Practices

For all tasks identified as falling into Categories I and II, the employer should have written procedures, and employees who perform these types of tasks should have ready access to those policies. Examples of written work practice procedures include things like safe collection and ultimate disposal of all body fluids and tissues in accordance with applicable local, state, and federal regulations. These written guidelines should also provide specific and detailed measures to be observed when handling sharp objects like needles, and puncture-resistant receptacles must be readily accessible for depositing such materials after use.

Personal Protective Equipment

The OSHA guidelines specify that the employer should provide and maintain personal protective equipment like gloves, masks, gowns, aprons, and face shields that are appropriate to the risk of exposure associated with each task. All Category I tasks do not involve the same type or degree of risk; therefore, all do not require the same kind or extent of protection. For example, paramedics responding to an auto accident might protect against cuts on metal and glass by wearing gloves or gauntlets that are both puncture resistant and impervious to blood. Such protective clothing must be provided for all employees performing Category I tasks, and workers performing Category II tasks should have ready access to appropriate protective equipment. Workers performing Category II tasks need not wear protective equipment at all times, but they should be prepared to use the equipment or clothing on short notice.

Medical Services

Because OSHA regulations apply to all bloodborne diseases, in addition to any health-care or medical surveillance required by other rules, regulations, or labor-management agreement, the employer should make available at no cost to the worker voluntary immunization against hepatitis B for all workers whose employment requires them to perform Category I tasks and who test negative for hepatitis B antibodies. If a worker tested positive for hepatitis B antibodies, the immunization would not be administered because the person is presumed to have already been infected. OSHA and CDC promote immunizations that may cost over $100 per employee, because AIDS and hepatitis B are transmitted to humans in the same way except that the virus that causes hepatitis B is far more infectious than the virus that causes AIDS. Because a proven, effective vaccine exists to combat hepatitis B, any worker performing Category I tasks (contact with blood and/or body secretions) should receive the immunization.

The second component of any medical services program in which Category I tasks are performed is to monitor, at the request of the worker, for the presence of HIV or hepatitis B antibodies following known or suspected occupational exposure to blood, body fluids, or tissues. In other words, if and when accidental exposures do occur, the employer is responsible for paying the costs associated with any testing the employee might undergo to ascertain if actual infection did occur as a result of the exposure. Such testing can be done by occupational health professionals, a private physician, or a county health department.

The third requirement of a medical service program for Category I workers is to provide medical counseling for all employees who are found to be seropositive for AIDS or hepatitis B antibodies as a result of a presumed occupational exposure. Medical counseling can be readily handled by the occupational health-care professional.

Recordkeeping

The last OSHA-specified responsibility of the employer of workers who perform either Category I or II tasks is to document procedures used to protect the worker from occupational exposure to bloodborne diseases. Therefore, the employer should maintain records documenting the administrative procedures used to classify job tasks, as well as the rationale for each task classification. For example, how many Category I or II workers are there, what specific Category I tasks are they likely to perform, and what measures have been taken to educate and provide the workers with protective equipment?

Additionally, copies of all written procedures, including the administrative review and approval process, should be readily accessible, as should training records that indicate the dates, content of training sessions, and names of persons conducting and receiving the training. Employee's compliance or noncompliance in using protective clothing and equipment should be periodically recorded, and the conditions associated with each incident of mucous membrane or skin exposure to body fluids or tissues must be carefully documented, as should the extant conditions and circumstances surrounding the incident. Finally, a description of any corrective measure taken to prevent a recurrence of a similar exposure should be documented.

Although CDC guidelines or universal precautions are in many ways self-explanatory, implementation in the worksite requires innovation, reeducation for lay first-aid providers, and a certain amount of retraining and orientation for the occupational health professional. Additionally, the work environment must be assessed for types of probable blood and body-fluid contact, and necessary equipment must be ordered and stored in readily accessible locations.

In worksites such as heavy industry where injuries and other medical emergencies are apt to occur, at least one member of every team or shift is designated as the first responder or the one who is trained in first-aid techniques. These individuals must be familiar with universal precautions, and they should be provided with needed equipment. Just as important is the fact that workers should be instructed to wash their hands or other skin surfaces thoroughly, should they become contaminated with someone else's blood.

Where certain workers are designated as first responders to provide on-site first aid, care providers should role-play situations in which they are required to select and don appropriate barrier equipment. Such practice sessions give workers an opportunity to become familiar with supplies like gloves and learn to deal with a decreased tactile sense when gloves are used.

The occupational health professional should also review the guidelines for prevention of HIV transmission in light of the actual characteristics of the routine and emergency care delivered in the workplace. Individual policies related to prevention of HIV transmission vary from one another in that each work setting has its own unique characteristics.

SUMMARY

Risk of occupational HIV infection is minimal but nonetheless a reality for health-care workers and others who come into contact with blood and body fluids as part of their job function. That risk is minimized by observation of universal precautions. The employer's responsibility revolves around identifying Category I and II employees and developing, implementing, and evaluating policies that guide employees' behavior, as well as seeing that needed protective equipment is purchased, utilized, and maintained properly.

REFERENCES

Centers for Disease Control (1988) Update: Universal precautions for prevention of transmission of human immunodeficiency virus, hepatitis B virus, and other bloodborne pathogens in health-care settings. *Morbidity and Mortality Weekly Report* 37(s-4):377–388.

Centers for Disease Control (1987) Recommendations for prevention of HIV transmission in health-care settings. *Morbidity and Mortality Weekly Report* 36(2s):1s–18s.

Department of Labor (1987) Joint advisory notice; Department of Labor; Department of Health and Human Services; HBV/HIV. *Federal Register* 52(210):41818–41823.

Tierno, P. M. (1988) AIDS overview: New guidelines for handling specimens. *American Journal of Continuing Education in Nursing* (special issue), 1–14.

Turner, J. G., H. J. Fawal, M. N. Long & M. P. Rivers (1988) Preventing HIV transmission in health-care settings. *American Association of Occupational Health Nurses Journal* 36(7):254–257.

10.
A PUBLIC RELATIONS AND MEDIA PERSPECTIVE

Public relations managers and other professionals in the corporate environment responsible for communicating policy to external audiences, either directly or through the media, are a company's frontline defense against the barrage of negative publicity that can result from a case of AIDS in the workplace.

The fully prepared public (PR) relations practitioner is a company's strongest link in minimizing the degree of crisis intervention normally needed to protect a firm's image when it becomes the subject of front-page headlines. However, a serious problem faces today's company PR or media relations professional.

While the AIDS epidemic continues to grow, most American businesses are still grappling with an answer for how to deal with AIDS in the workplace. The overwhelming majority refuse

This chapter was written by Charles B. Michelini, Senior Science Writer, University of Alabama at Birmingham.

to develop an AIDS policy until they are confronted with a case of the disease in their worker population. A recent *Fortune* magazine and Allstate Insurance survey of 600 American firms revealed most do not deal with the issue until they absolutely have to—when an employee is stricken with AIDS (AIDS: Corporate America, 1988). This denial or reality avoidance naturally puts the company's public relations representative in the most precarious of positions.

More than half of those surveyed in the Fortune-Allstate study reported they felt an image problem would result if the public were to find out that someone in their company had AIDS. Some of the actions executives said they would take are probably illegal. Nevertheless, today's proactive CEOs in major companies and those at the helm of small and midsize firms cannot afford to duck the issue.

At one time or another, every company will have to resolve these basic questions: Should employees be screened for AIDS? Who is going to pay for a worker's medical care if he or she contracts AIDS? What is management doing to educate workers regarding the spread of AIDS? The public relations representative who does not have concrete answers will ultimately take the heat in-house.

Going a step further, companies should recognize the potential negative media and public relations implications when faced with the following dilemmas:

- What if an employee refuses to work next to an AIDS patient or someone who has a positive HIV-antibody test?
- How will the company respond when the confidentiality of an employee with AIDS is violated?
- How will the company respond to discrimination charges if it is accused of refusing to hire a person who has AIDS or a positive HIV-antibody test?
- Can the company fire an employee with AIDS?
- How is the company going to respond to rumors of an employee with AIDS?

Because much of what the public relations department will impart to the media and other audiences will rely heavily, if not exclusively, on corporate AIDS policy, the PR professional has to call management's attention to the lack of policy. In the most open environments, this advice will be met with gratitude; in many companies, however, middle and lower-level management will hesitate to broach the subject with their superiors. This reluctance is understandable but counterproductive because most company spokespersons will at some time be asked substantive questions regarding a case of AIDS in the workplace. Lack of policy will probably elicit reactionary, defensive responses to media and public inquiries. These types of responses, as knowledgeable media specialists realize, impart a negative impression. Assuming that the PR department's mission is to help put the firm's best foot forward, a proactive stance is almost always the desirable mode of action.

Dwayne Summar, president of the Public Relations Society of America (PRCA), puts it this way: "The PR practitioner is needed to help solve the [company's] dilemma. With this crucial health issue we can deliver the message that by addressing AIDS in the workplace a company is not only assisting employees, but will actually gain better public relations when AIDS enters their workplace." (American Red Cross, 1988, p.6)

After all, AIDS has hit every area of the country. No employer can afford to believe his or her company and its employees are immune. Some businesses may have had the luxury of not yet dealing with this issue, but deal with it they will. Just one case can totally disrupt an organization, and smaller firms that feel they will never be touched by the disease and its subsequent public, media, and human relations fallout are the most vulnerable.

Remember, in today's instant news environment, national stories initiate from all over the country. A company in the Deep South can have an in-house AIDS crisis at 5 P.M. and find itself spotlighted on the 6 o'clock news from Buffalo to Boise. It will not have weeks to prepare an approach to the problem.

The company spokesperson must be immediately ready to answer the tough questions to gain the media's confidence.

THE MEDIA

As most spokespersons are aware, every time a firm's name is attached to a controversial issue it becomes a potential "story" in the local, regional, or national press. In the last decade, no public health issue has garnered more media coverage than the AIDS crisis. Because of this, editors continue to demand copy from reporters, and the reporters' responsibility is to seek out stories and report on issues that may impact on the community. Certainly a case of AIDS, particularly in companies located in small to midsize communities, is newsworthy if controversy is at its center.

Historically, AIDS began as an infectious disease curiosity in the early 1980s, but rapidly picked up momentum (see Figure 10-1). This was due, in part, to the increasing number of celebrities, such as Rock Hudson, who died of the disease. The AIDS epidemic will not go away, and even the most optimistic projections put the target date for a viable vaccine at somewhere around the turn of the century.

Given the fact that more than 78,000 cases of AIDS have been reported in the United States, and more than half of them have died, by 1991 everyone in the country will know someone who has been directly affected by AIDS, and many of them will be someone's coworker. If an event was ever worthy of day-to-day coverage from the media's perspective, it is AIDS. The media may not be far off the mark either, according to summaries of national public opinion surveys on AIDS from 1983 through 1986 (Blake & Arkin, 1988).

The data reveal that by June 1983, 77 percent of respondents in one poll and 81 percent in another reported having heard something about AIDS. Polls conducted in July and August of 1983 found the percentage had increased to 91 percent. By 1985, responses to the same question suggested

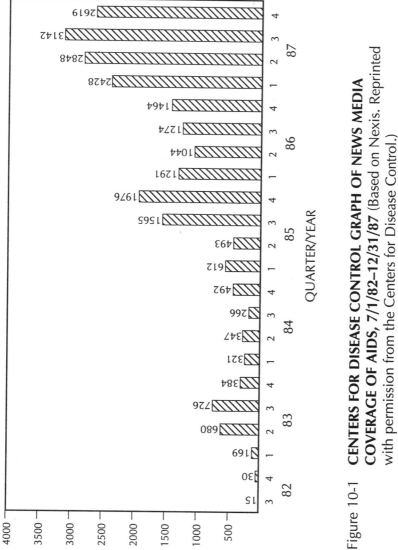

Figure 10-1 **CENTERS FOR DISEASE CONTROL GRAPH OF NEWS MEDIA COVERAGE OF AIDS, 7/1/82–12/31/87** (Based on Nexis. Reprinted with permission from the Centers for Disease Control.)

151

that 95 percent to 97 percent of the American public had heard or read something about AIDS. More than half the 1985 respondents (58 percent) replied that they had heard or read "a lot" about the disease, and an additional 30 percent reported having heard or read some information about the disease.

When queried about their specific exposure to news in the media, nearly 25 percent said they paid more attention to stories about AIDS than any other topic. Twenty-four percent said they had encountered seven stories about AIDS in the media during the past week, and 82 percent responded that they had seen at least two stories. Clearly, in 1985, high levels of media exposure were paralleled by high levels of expressed public interest in AIDS relative to other items in the news. Beyond 1989, the trend is likely to continue.

Other 1985 polls explored public opinion regarding the quality and quantity of the media's coverage of AIDS and AIDS-related issues. When asked how the print media and television had handled AIDS, 55 percent of the general public replied "about right," 21 percent indicated too much coverage, and 16 percent said not enough. Most respondents (59 percent) did not think the press had exaggerated the health risk of AIDS, but 34 percent did. Sixty percent felt strongly or somewhat strongly that the "hysteria over AIDS" was, for the most part, created by the media. Twenty-nine percent of respondents thought AIDS had been handled too delicately in the media (see Table 10-2).

Combining the revelations of the polls mentioned above with a fair measure of common sense, we can safely assume that we would have to search far and wide across the vast expanse of America's labor force before encountering an individual who does not have at least a casual interest in AIDS.

That much interest in any topic spells news, particularly when the subject reaches into the workplace. From the media's perspective, which is entirely realistic in this case, AIDS in the work environment is a multidimensional concern because it cuts across matters of policy, medicine, social responsibility, economics, labor relations, and ethics. With that in mind, media relations practitioners in businesses large and small ought to begin asking themselves: "What do I do when my company becomes the news?"

Few public relations or media relations professionals would argue the nightmarish implications behind the following headlines:

EMPLOYEES WALK OFF JOB,
REFUSE TO WORK WITH AIDS PATIENT

DEAD MAN'S LAST WORDS:
THE COMPANY KILLED ME

SECRETARY WITH AIDS SUES BOSS

XYZ TESTS FOR AIDS WITHOUT PERMISSION

DISCRIMINATION LEVELED
AGAINST FAST-FOOD CAFE

Effective public relations forecasting and action can often reduce or avoid serious damage, and employee education from the top down is the first step.

THE BASICS OF CORPORATE AIDS COMMUNICATION

During a recent informal gathering of several journalists who routinely report on AIDS for local, regional, and national publications, including the *New York Times,* the *Los Angeles Times* syndicate, the *Chicago Tribune*, the *Miami Herald,* the *Birmingham News* and others, a recurring theme echoed around the room: "I'm tired of the same old flack from company PRs. They keep saying they treat AIDS like any other catastrophic illness. If that's the case, how come John Doe gets fired for a minor infraction of a rule or some other lame excuse because he has AIDS, yet others in the company with cancer or heart disease aren't discriminated against. I just don't buy it."

By now most reporters who routinely deal with AIDS are not buying the party line either. They have come in direct contact with AIDS patients and realize the devastating nature of the

Table 10-1 **RESPONSES TO 1985 PUBLIC OPINION POLLS REGARDING MEDIA COVERAGE OF AIDS**

CBS NEWS/NEW YORK TIMES POLL OF 762 ADULTS:		*LOS ANGELES TIMES* POLL OF 2,308 ADULTS:	
How do you think the press and TV have handled the AIDS story?		Is the "hysteria over AIDS" largely a media creation?	
Too much of it	21%	Agree strongly	30%
Not enough	16%	Agree somewhat	30%
About right	55%	Disagree somewhat	20%
Don't know/No answer	8%	Disagree strongly	15%
		Not sure	5%
		Have the media exaggerated the health risks?	
		Yes	34%
		No	59%
		Not sure	7%
		Have the media handled AIDS too delicately or avoided specifics?	
		Yes	29%
		No	61%
		Not sure	9%
		Refused	1%

Note. From *AIDS Information Monitor* by S. Blake and E. Arken, 1988, American Red Cross. Reprinted with permission of the American Red Cross.

disease. They *do* get involved. If the company has problems with its workforce or public image, many believe, maybe the company has not done its part in communicating the facts to employees and its various other constituencies.

In the 1988 volume *AIDS: Corporate America Responds,* the Allstate Forum on Public Issues points out that by bringing the facts about AIDS to employees and their families, companies can play a major role in educating the public, and thus help to control the spread of the disease and allay irrational fears.

> Some people may question the need for a corporate AIDS program or policy; after all, there isn't one for Alzheimer's disease or cancer. But as we all know, AIDS is not just a medical condition, it is also a social and cultural phenomenon. If we are to control and ultimately prevail over it, a collective national effort is needed, and the business community has a key role to play. Whether a company has an AIDS program or not, it will still need to be prepared for employees who are affected by the AIDS virus; the attitudes of, and effects on, their co-workers; as well as possible litigation or negative publicity (*AIDS: Corporate America*, 1988, p. 56).

Although no one person, function, or department should be charged with developing an AIDS policy, the general consensus is that the public relations arm of an organization should be involved in spearheading the project. Public relations must be involved from the outset and interface directly with the CEO, the human relations or personnel manager, and the firm's legal and medical staffs.

Elsewhere in this text the basic procedures of setting up appropriate internal communications through policy and education are addressed (see chapters 3 and 5), and some of the same devices apply to external audiences. Many of the following suggestions for communicating with external audiences were adapted from information provided through *AIDS: A Matter of Corporate Policy,* a national interactive video conference held in May 1988. Other portions are a combination of the author's recommendations and those made during the Allstate Forum on Public Issues.

COMMUNICATING WITH EXTERNAL AUDIENCES

Companies wishing to go on record as taking a proactive stance on AIDS should consider communicating with external audiences before the firm is put on the defensive. These external audiences may include, but are not limited to, customers, suppliers, community groups, shareholders, public officials, media, the financial community, AIDS groups, and other organizations who have shown an interest in AIDS.

Media

When the firm decides to put an AIDS education program in place, communicate it to the local media. Let local print and broadcast outlets know that the company is aware of the controversial nature of the subject, yet that it wishes to do everything in its power to educate the community and help curb the incidence of the disease. Go on record now as a leader rather than a follower. The firm can usually expect positive widespread publicity through the local print and broadcast media if it comes out up front.

Local Business Community

Consider addressing a letter from the firm's CEO or other appropriate executive to local business leaders encouraging top-level management to initiate, or at least consider, AIDS workplace programs.

Once the company has made a decision to address the AIDS issue in the workplace, approach the local Chamber of Commerce and investigate the possibilities of that organization, in conjunction with the company and a local public health agency, cosponsoring seminars on the subject. Once the majority of businesses come out in the open, the normal paranoia usually associated with the issue will begin to diminish. If a seminar or workshop seems inappropriate, try a breakfast or luncheon meeting with key business leaders.

Those firms located in areas where AIDS has not become a local issue might want to consider forming a corporate coalition. Such a partnership with other area firms could help support advertising and public information programs and act on behalf of all member businesses.

One proactive tactic employed by several companies is to make a public contribution to a service or other health-care organization that is dealing with AIDS. This action can help to ease the firm into an area it heretofore has avoided. The recipient of the donation and the company can issue simultaneous press releases announcing the contribution.

Encourage the firm's CEO to write a letter to the editor of the local newspaper highlighting why business must become involved with helping stem the AIDS epidemic. Tailor the letter to fit comfortably with community attitudes, but stick with the facts. Always stress that AIDS is *not* a disease confined to the homosexual and intravenous drug-abusing communities and that it cannot be transmitted by casual contact.

WHERE TO GET HELP WITH PUBLIC RELATIONS

Even the most experienced practitioner may need help in relating to the public and the media on the issue of AIDS in the workplace. For this reason the Public Relations Society of America and the American Red Cross recently joined forces and developed materials that offer guidance to public relations

professionals and businesses in general. The educational programs offered by the Red Cross, combined with the communications expertise of PRSA members located in virtually every
geographical area of the country, can provide the guidance
needed to take that first step. Although other resources are
available for implementing an AIDS education program (see
Appendix E), the special needs of the media relations specialist
or public relations manager will probably be most expeditiously met through the Red Cross-PRSA partnership.

A final note. What follows is a case study, which was originally published under the title "Panic Prevention—Educating
Employees about AIDS," in the *Public Relations Journal*. Although what appears below is only a portion of the original
article, some PR practitioners have found it a useful tool when
directed to the attention of their CEO.

> Many organizations are finding that a comprehen-
> sive education program for co-workers can halt the
> hysteria about AIDS in the workplace.
>
> Paul Cronan reported for work on October 21, but
> it was not just a day like any other. Cronan, an
> installer/repairer at a Needham, Massachusetts ga-
> rage at New England Telephone, was returning to
> work as part of an out-of-court settlement of a dis-
> crimination/breach-of-privacy lawsuit, a suit he had
> filed because he had AIDS. New England Telephone
> had hoped Cronan's return would mark a period,
> ending an ugly chapter in its employee relations;
> instead it was merely a comma.
>
> Other employees in the Needham garage were un-
> comfortable with Cronan's presence his first day
> back, and the air was abuzz with questions of
> whether they could catch the disease from him. On
> the second day, two-thirds of the employees refused
> to come to work. Scrambling to resolve the crisis,
> New England Telephone rounded up physicians
> from Massachusetts General Hospital, who, together

with their in-house medical experts, held an evening seminar about AIDS. Employees of the garage, spouses and family members crowded in to get the facts. Thus the crisis ended; employees returned to work the following day.

Unfortunately, New England Telephone is not alone. As AIDS whirls across the country a second epidemic—panic—is getting caught in its winds, a problem particularly affecting the workplace. Stricken employees returning to work are sometimes greeted by what amounts to a lynch mob.

Most worksites have so far been spared this employee-relations megacrisis. But experts say the current number of AIDS cases in the U.S. is merely the flurries before the storm, so the problem will strike many organizations in the coming years. Some of the larger employers in the highest-case cities of New York, San Francisco and Los Angeles have begun to develop employee-education programs to help allay co-workers' fears, say experts, that are medically unfounded. Other organizations, however, have not yet even begun to address the issue.

"AIDS may be the biggest issue in the San Francisco area," says Al Ellison, community relations director at Pacific Bell, which is headquartered there. "So companies here are forced to deal with it. That's not the case in other areas of the country. AIDS may not even be on their Top 10 list."

Many say that it ought to be. "Without doubt, fear of contracting the disease can cause considerable disruption ... in the workplace," the American Management Association notes in its monograph, AIDS: The Workplace Issues. The September 1987 issue of *Across the Board*, a magazine for top executives published by the Conference Board, tells of a financial company facing the return of an AIDS-stricken employee; one supervisor, who had been with the company for years, was so adamant in her refusal to work around the man that she ultimately quit her job.

When an employee is known to have—or just suspected of having—AIDS, co-workers' concerns about the spread of the disease can turn to hysterics. Company after company report that employees have refused to work with or touch that person, or use the same bathroom, telephone, water fountain or pencil. One AIDS victim was not even allowed to use his pregnant co-worker's word processor; she claimed she had once seen him sweat on the keyboard.

"It's been obvious that those companies not dealing with the AIDS issue (who then have an employee coming down with it) have seen smooth functioning of the workplace disabled," says Tom White, marketing manager of the San Francisco AIDS Foundation, a non-profit organization set up to deal with AIDS.

In addition to preventing panic, many say, education in the workplace can help halt the spread of the disease. "Adults spend a majority of their time in the workplace," says White. "It's effective to educate them there." Surgeon General C. Everett Koop, M.D., has also called for education in the workplace. As yet there is no cure for AIDS, he says, but the disease "is preventable. With proper information and education, as many as 12,000 to 14,000 people could be saved in 1991," he says.

"Companies need to think about AIDS," says Jim Foley, manager of media relations at Pacific Bell. Pacific Bell decided a few years ago that it needed an employee-education program because employees, who were reading about AIDS in the local press, started grilling their supervisors about the workplace risks—before any employee had even been diagnosed with AIDS (there have been several since).

Koop recently recommended that all companies begin to educate employees before the first such case appears at the worksite. "To wait for an employee to develop AIDS is a time bomb," says Philip Pagano, director of employee communications at the American Medical Association. "At that point, there's not as much credibility; it could look like the company is covering up." Companies need to educate employees about the disease, Pagano says, and about what's expected of them, so that "when—not if—an employee develops AIDS there won't be as many problems," he adds, noting that most sizeable employers are going to have to deal with AIDS in their organization sooner or later.

Unfortunately, statistics bear Pagano out. The number of AIDS cases in the U.S. has virtually doubled every year since 1981. To date, 78,000 cases (revised for 1988) have been reported (56 percent of stricken adults have since died). If the present rate of infection continues, the Centers for Disease Control expects the disease will claim 270,000 by 1991. Perhaps more important in terms of the disease's spread, an estimated 1.5 million seemingly healthy Americans have been exposed to the virus but show no symptoms; all of these carriers are thought to be able to pass the disease (estimates range from 10 to 50 percent for the number of this group who will develop full-blown AIDS). Today almost half of all cases come from New York, San Francisco and Los Angeles—though AIDS has been reported in all 50 states—but experts expect by 1991 fully 80 percent will come from elsewhere.

The national media have given AIDS substantial coverage since the disease was first detected in 1981. But new articles, such as the *Atlantic*'s recent cover story, "Heterosexuals and AIDS: The Second

Stage of the Epidemic," and *U.S. News & World Report's* "AIDS: At the Dawn of Fear," chronicle the spread of the disease into the non-drug-abusing heterosexual population. (While 9 out of 10 cases nationwide continue to occur in homosexual men and those who inject abused drugs, the percentage of heterosexually transmitted cases has recently doubled to 4 percent in total.) Articles like these are bound to raise a new round of concern among people who had believed their lives would be untouched by AIDS, and now fear that a co-worker—or the co-worker's husband, aunt or neighbor—may have it. Most professionals involved with the issue say that an education program for employees often needs to start with upper management. "The person whose education is most important is the CEO, whose understanding of AIDS is essential to receiving the authority and resources needed to do the job and do it well," said W. Harry Brownlee, M.D., a counselor to companies' employee assistance program, at a forum on AIDS sponsored by the New York Business Group on Health in 1986. "Managers and executives may in some instances be more urbane and sophisticated, but their need for AIDS education may be no less than that of employees on the lower levels," he said.

Upper management must be taught about how AIDS is spread, about the law regarding employee confidentiality—unless the employee agrees, not even his supervisor can be told (part of Cronan's suit, in fact, was based on this breach of privacy)—and the legal issues. White suggests that middle management and outside consultants take a strong position when dealing with the top brass. "Top managers are recalcitrant to take on the issue. It may help your position if you use other companies as examples of successful efforts," he advises. ("Panic Prevention" by Meryl Davids. Reprinted from the March 1987 issue of the *Public Relations Journal*, with permission of the Public Relations Society of America, copyright 1987.)

SUMMARY

What a public relations professional can say to the media and to other groups is dependent on the corporate AIDS policy and the company's efforts to educate its employees. Remember that spokespersons are best prepared to answer media questions when the company has done its homework on the inevitable issues surrounding AIDS.

REFERENCES

American Red Cross (1988) PRSA/American Red Cross partnership-AIDS education in the workplace (Script and Video available from the American Red Cross, National Headquarters, 17th & D Streets NW, Washington, DC 20006).

AIDS: Corporate America Responds. A Report of Corporate Involvement (1988) New York: Allstate Insurance Co.

Blake, S. M., & Arkin, E. B. (1988) *AIDS Information Monitor: A Summary of National Public Opinion Surveys on AIDS 1983–1986.* Washington, DC: American National Red Cross.

Davids, M. (1987) Panic prevention. *Public Relations Journal* 11(3):18.

Engel, P. G. (1986) When AIDS struck: Two firms' responses might be role models. *Industry Week* (May 12) 18–19.

Halcrow, A. (1986) AIDS: The corporate response. *Personnel* 65(6):123–127.

Herold, D. M. (1988) *Employees' Reactions to AIDS in the Workplace.* Atlanta: Georgia Institute of Technology.
Letchinger, R. S. (1987) AIDS: An employer's dilemma. *Personnel* 7(1):58–63.

11.

APPROACHES TO PREVENTION AND CONTROL OF AIDS

What action must we take today to assure the prevention and control of AIDS? What is being done by the federal government to contain this dreaded disease? Although education has been touted as the major strategy for reducing the spread of AIDS, a multifaceted public health approach to prevention has already been implemented in this country. This massive public health approach includes education, risk assessments, voluntary and mandatory risk counseling and testing, contact tracing and reporting, protecting the nation's blood supply, vaccine development, and distribution of condoms and sterile needles. The intent of this chapter is to describe the progress that has been made on each of these preventive fronts in our efforts to combat AIDS.

EDUCATION

Responding to AIDS as a major public health crisis in the United States, the federal government has been most visible in terms of public education efforts. The National AIDS Information and Education Program (NAIEP) was established within the Centers for Disease Control (CDC) in April 1987. The purpose of this program is to centralize HIV public information and education efforts within CDC. NAIEP received $23.6 million in 1987 and $41 million in 1988 in operating budget to conduct the following major activities:

1. The National AIDS Information Campaign. This media-based information campaign is intended to communicate HIV information to the American public. A large public relations firm received the $7.9 million contract to influence positively knowledge and attitudes regarding AIDS. Frequent public service announcements in the media are part of this effort. The most notable accomplishment of the campaign was a mailing of the 8-page "Understanding AIDS" brochure to 100 million households in 1988.
2. The National AIDS Clearinghouse. The federal government proposes to serve as a resource center for all HIV materials. Free brochures in large or small quantity can be obtained from the Clearinghouse (see Appendix E). A total of $2.2 million was awarded for this activity in 1988.
3. The National AIDS Hotline. The Public Health Service toll-free hotline, (800) 342-AIDS, provides callers with recorded general information about AIDS. A toll-free number is also provided for individuals with specific questions about AIDS and the location of AIDS-antibody testing sites.
4. A minority outreach program. Through a grants and contract mechanism, NAIEP administers a minority outreach program to assist national and regional organizations in targeting information to minority populations. Funding for FY 1988 was $19.5 million ("Commission Says," 1988).

In June 1988, President Reagan's Commission on the Human Immunodeficiency Virus Epidemic reported its findings of deficiencies in the nation's response to AIDS. In particular, lack of funding and lack of personnel within CDC were cited, and over 500 recommendations were presented. As a result of this report, a major revision in federal policy was anticipated within months of the end of the Reagan administration ("Reagan Seeks New AIDS Policies," 1988).

RISK ASSESSMENT

As a further preventive effort in this country, all health professionals in public and private sectors have been urged to provide AIDS education and to help individuals assess their risk for AIDS. Companies, schools, and community organizations have joined in this effort. CDC Director James Mason identified the workplace as an excellent site for educating adults and further stated that companies have a responsibility for assisting their employees to maintain health and eliminate risky behaviors (Stein, 1987).

Clearly, agreement exists on the segments of the population who are at high risk and on what behaviors are high risk. High-risk groups include individuals who have engaged in male homosexual activity or IV drug use in the last 10 years, persons who have resided in Haiti or Central Africa, male or female prostitutes, hemophiliacs and persons with a history of multiple blood transfusions, newborn infants of high-risk or infected mothers, and individuals who have had a sex partner in one of the high-risk groups (Benza & Zumwalde, 1986; Hearst & Hulley, 1988). High-risk behaviors include unprotected sexual acts with persons of unknown or high risk and sharing needles with infected persons. Epidemiologic investigations demonstrate that the HIV virus is transmitted by sex, blood, and mother-to-child routes.

The following precautions are recommended in order to reduce risk of exposure to the HIV virus:

1. Have sex only with persons who are at low risk for exposure to HIV. Mutually monogamous relationships over the past 10 years and abstinence are the best means of avoiding exposure. Listen for information about a partner's past history and ask directly about risk status before the relationship develops into a sexual one. Avoid sex with anyone who is seropositive or who is in a high-risk group unless they have discontinued high-risk activities for at least 6 months and have later had a negative HIV screening test, the ELISA (Hearst & Hulley, 1988).
2. Use latex condoms with a spermicidal (contraceptive) jelly containing nonoxynol-9 if your sex partner's risk status is unknown or if the relationship has not been mutually monogamous for a long term. Latex condoms when used properly seem to be effective in blocking the transmission of the virus. In addition, spermicidal jelly has been shown to kill the AIDS virus in laboratory experiments. If a lubricant is also used, only a water-based lubricant such as K-Y jelly is recommended because oil-based lubricants including petroleum jelly, vegetable shortening, and mineral oil weaken the rubber in condoms within minutes ("Next to Abstinence," 1988).
3. Avoid sex with multiple partners because of the increased risk of exposure to someone with HIV.
4. Avoid the use of illicit drugs, alcohol, barbiturates, amphetamines, and other substances that reduce your ability to control high-risk sexual behaviors (Christ & Wiener, 1985).
5. Postpone pregnancy if you or your partner are in a high-risk group.
6. Have HIV testing before planning a pregnancy if you and your partner have not been in mutually monogamous relationship for the past ten years (Hearst & Hulley, 1988).
7. Do not share IV needles and syringes if you use drugs. Only

sterile equipment can protect you from the HIV virus.
8. If planning elective surgery in which blood transfusion may be needed, contact your local hospital to inquire about autologous transfusion, that is, banking your own blood for use at the time of surgery.

Gay organizations have been effective in publicizing the need for risk assessments among homosexual and bisexual men. The spread of AIDS among these groups and among unknowing female partners of bisexual men hopefully has been reduced because of safer sex practices.

Preventing HIV infection among drug users and their sexual partners is a much more difficult endeavor. Infected IV drug users are responsible for most of the heterosexual and perinatal (to newborns) transmission of AIDS. In New York City, IV drug users account for almost 87 percent of the heterosexual transmission and 80 percent of the infant cases of AIDS (DesJarlais & Friedman, 1988). Sharing of needles and syringes is the mode of transmission of the HIV virus among IV drug users. Halting the spread of AIDS in this group will necessitate decreasing illegal drug use in this country, expanding drug-treatment programs, teaching IV drug users sterilization procedures, and providing sterile disposable needles and syringes. Already reports from New York tell about how the increased demand for sterile needles has prompted sellers on the street to rewrap and sell dirty needles as though they were sterile (Institute of Medicine, 1986a). In some cities, outreach efforts have been used to teach IV drug users to use bleach and other methods to sterilize injection equipment. In most locations, the demand for treatment in drug programs is greater than the availability of treatment; therefore, resources for drug rehabilitation are limited. The threat of AIDS will be unlikely to persuade IV drug users to discontinue drug use. Therefore, the preventive approach with the most potential for success among IV drug users is that of providing sterile needles and syringes.

Another population that appears to warrant risk assessment is the adolescent group. The adolescent years are often a time of experimentation with sex and drugs (Institute of Medicine, 1986a). We are already aware that 57 percent of all adolescents are sexually active by age 17 and that 40 percent of teen-age girls become pregnant at least once by age 20 (Kibrick, 1988). Teenagers must be thoroughly educated about the risk of AIDS, encouraged to abstain from sex, and, if sexually active, encouraged to practice safer sex.

RISK-REDUCTION COUNSELING AND TESTING

Public health officials have also utilized risk-reduction counseling and testing to control the AIDS epidemic (see Appendix C for U.S. Public Health Service Guidelines for Testing and Counseling). Voluntary anonymous counseling and HIV-antibody testing of high-risk groups has been available at federally designated test sites throughout the country. Pre- and post-test counseling is required for all persons who are tested at these sites. Persons in high-risk groups are encouraged to take advantage of the services. HIV counseling and testing programs are needed for the following reasons:

1. To monitor the epidemic and plan public health control measures
2. To identify individuals who are seropositive so that they may change sex and drug behaviors and thus reduce the spread of infection
3. To alert individuals to signs and symptoms of AIDS so that diagnosis and treatment can begin early
4. To identify individuals who would be candidates for medications currently under investigation as treatments for AIDS (Institute of Medicine, 1986b).

The question of mandatory HIV testing and counseling for the general population and for high-risk groups has generally had unfavorable reviews. In practical terms, to monitor the disease effectively, HIV testing would have to be conducted on large numbers every 6 months. Premarital testing, although proposed as a mandatory screening program, would be costly and low in yield. Of the 2.5 million marriages per year or 5 million persons to be tested, only approximately 250 infected females and 1,000 infected males would be identified as HIV-antibody positive, and this at a cost of about $200 million (Chin, 1988). Testing high-risk groups such as homosexual and bisexual men, IV drug users, prostitutes, prisoners, and pregnant women can be fraught with problems ranging from discrimination to invasion of private consensual behavior.

Only in prisons, mental institutions, homes for the mentally retarded, and the military has mandatory AIDS testing been considered justifiable. Authorities of these institutions and organizations have a legal obligation to prevent the spread of infections within those facilities (Institute of Medicine, 1986b). The military argues for mandatory HIV testing to protect immunocompromised persons who may be at greater risk when stationed in foreign lands with high disease rates and to protect them from the live virus vaccinations required of all new recruits. Other reasons for HIV testing in the military are that seropositive individuals would be unable to provide blood for transfusions during emergencies and that the military needs to minimize the risks of transmitting AIDS to sexual partners in other countries where military personnel are stationed.

Compulsory measures such as isolation and quarantine, which are often used to prevent the spread of communicable diseases, have been suggested in the media and in legislatures in this country. These means have been rejected because those dying from AIDS do not present as great a threat as the more than one million asymptomatic HIV-antibody-positive persons who are carriers of the infection. To conduct mass-screening programs to identify and isolate these individuals would infringe on civil liberties. In a few instances, recalcitrant individuals, such as infected prostitutes who continue to endanger others, have been court sentenced to house confinement. Because HIV infectivity is lifelong, house confinement can only be a temporary, ineffective measure. Not only must we encourage those who are infected to protect others from AIDS as their moral obligation but also individuals such as prostitutes may need to have job training or confinement to a hospital or hospice where they work for room and board (Eldridge, 1988). Men and women must be educated that anonymous sex is dangerous (Wolfsy, 1988).

From a legal standpoint, judges ruling on drug abuse and prostitution cases may use the court's power to require that these high-risk individuals have HIV testing and counseling. The attorney general in Georgia rendered an opinion that judges can require HIV testing just as they already require prostitutes to be tested for sexually transmitted diseases (Eldridge, 1988).

Compulsory closings of some New York City and San Francisco bathhouses and bars has also been a last-resort public health measure (Institute of Medicine, 1986b). Although public health officers have the authority to close any facility that may endanger the public's health, such closings have occurred only after regulatory inspections and requests that proprietors discourage high-risk sexual behaviors. In these facilities, the operators were blatantly encouraging high-risk behavior in the face of a growing public health epidemic.

REPORTING AND CONTACT TRACING

Other public health measures typically used to control communicable diseases include reporting and contact tracing. Every state requires that AIDS cases be promptly reported to the health department, which then reports the cases to CDC. Reporting is essential for epidemiologic surveillance of an epidemic. Only a few states, among them Colorado, Alabama and South Carolina, require reporting of names of cases so that contact tracing is possible. Proponents argue for these approaches because educational programs alone are not sufficient to control the epidemic. Those opposed to reporting and contact tracing voice concerns that high-risk individuals will avoid voluntary testing because they fear possible loss of confidentiality (Institute of Medicine, 1986a). On June 13, 1988, four medical societies in New York filed suit to force the New York State Department of Health to categorize AIDS as a communicable disease and begin contact tracing. The state health commissioner, David Axelrod, opposes the classification and believes that it will result in quarantines and drive the problem underground ("New York Medical Societies Sue," 1988).

Colorado, the first state to implement a program of reporting with some contact tracing, enters test results on a computer that is equipped with a security system and a system for follow-up notification. Although Colorado is a low-incidence state, the advocates for reporting maintain that they must track the incidence of HIV infection and provide counseling and a mechanism for contacting infected individuals when effective therapy becomes available (Institute of Medicine, 1986b).

In states with reporting and contact tracing, laboratories are required to report the name, address, and physician of all individuals with HIV-positive antibody results. Health department professionals then interview individuals with positive results, suggest that they notify their contacts, and request names of sexual partners and persons with whom they have shared needles. Contacts are offered screening tests and risk-reduction education and counseling. Thus public health officials pursue all avenues for controlling the epidemic. Although contact tracing may be preferred by those with a public health orientation, difficulties do arise because of the lengthy period between infection and diagnosis of disease, lack of treatment for contacts, and the potential for negative consequences for those identified (Institute of Medicine, 1986b).

PROTECTING THE NATION'S BLOOD SUPPLY

Early on in the AIDS epidemic, this bloodborne disease's threat to blood and tissue banking became evident. The first national effort to control AIDS was in the blood service area (Pindyck, 1987). Three major blood-banking organizations in this country, the American National Red Cross, the American

Association of Blood Banks, and the Council of Community Centers, are responsible for supplying 3 million patients per year with whole blood and blood components such as red blood cells, platelets, and factor 8, which is given to hemophiliacs. In a concerted effort, the Food and Drug Administration and the pharmaceutical industry rushed to develop an HIV-antibody screening test. This test, used in all blood-collection agencies since 1985, annually accounts for more than 20 million tests for HIV antibody. The public needs to be continually reassured that all blood donors are screened and all blood supplies are tested. In addition the public needs to be informed that no one can catch AIDS from being a blood donor.

Current procedures in the blood service organizations exclude potential donors at high risk for AIDS. Prospective donors are informed of high risk groups and are asked not to give blood if they are a member of one of the following groups:

1. Haitians who have entered the United States since 1977
2. Males who have had sexual contact with another male since 1977
3. IV drug users in the past or present
4. Hemophiliacs
5. Males or females who have had sexual contact with anyone in the above groups

Self-deferral is also encouraged by a privacy option. Because people are urged to give blood by friends, family, or coworkers, some donors may be reticent to admit that they are in a high-risk group. Therefore, a number of blood centers have developed a form on which the blood donor can indicate in a privacy booth whether the blood should be used for transfusion or should be used only for research purposes. The need for self-deferral is apparent because most recent seropositive donors were found to be members of high-risk groups, and false-negative results can occur because of the long period from HIV infection to the appearance of antibodies (Institute of Medicine, 1986b).

After blood is donated, the ELISA test for antibodies is performed. If the ELISA is positive on two or more tests of the blood specimen, a Western blot analysis is performed. The donor is notified only if the Western blot analysis confirms the presence of HIV antibodies. Seropositive donors are listed with local and national deferral registries to alert blood collection agencies not to accept subsequent donations, and the blood donation is discarded. Some blood centers notify seropositive donors and provide follow-up counseling.

To protect the blood supply, the threshold for the ELISA test has been set very low. Because the test is extremely sensitive in order to detect the presence of antibodies, it also sometimes results in false positives; that is, people who are not infected will sometimes test positive. The numbers of false positives greatly outnumbers the number of true positives in the blood-collection agencies because high-risk people are asked not to give blood (Institute of Medicine, 1986b). Any blood sample that tests positive in the blood banks is probably a false positive.

The "community responsibility" concept regarding blood donations prevails today. Although 25 percent of the donors during the 1970s were paid, 99 percent of the donors were volunteers in the 1980s (Holland, 1987). In some instances, blood donation was thought to be an individual's responsibility; that is, individuals were encouraged to get friends and family to donate blood for them. Questions have arisen as to whether blood from designated donors is as safe as blood from a screened community supply and as to whether family members who refuse to give blood will be suspected of being in a high-risk group. Another concern is whether designated donors would hold their blood "in reserve" in case a family member or friend would need it. All in all, the consensus is that directed donations are not favorable.

The safest blood source is oneself. Autologous donation, or banking one's own blood for later transfusion, is to be encouraged for all patients undergoing elective surgery. Surgeons and patients alike should plan ahead for autodonation so that patients can avoid all risks of both AIDS and hepatitis infections. Blood-banking organizations admit that autologous donations are the safest form of transfusion; however, they have not taken a lead in promoting this approach (Holland, 1987). Another mechanism under investigation is artificial blood and blood components. In the future a major company such as DuPont or Baxter-Travenol will no doubt produce these blood products to be administered in hospitals. Blood-collection agencies will not be involved with artificial blood products and therefore have little to gain in promoting this alternative.

THE PROMISE OF A VACCINE

Although HIV vaccines are in the developmental stages, an approved vaccine may not be available for years (Koff & Hoth, 1988; MacDonald, 1986). In fact, the barriers to development of a vaccine are so great that immunization cannot be viewed as a solution for the near future.

Among the difficulties in vaccine development is lack of current knowledge regarding mechanisms of protective immunity to the HIV virus. Antibodies produced from immunization may not be sufficient to protect people from HIV infection. The HIV virus also has a high mutation rate, which impedes progress in vaccine development. Most vaccines consist of live, attenuated (weakened) viruses and in the case of the HIV virus, the "possibility of the virus regaining its capacity to cause disease" is a great risk (Institute of Medicine, 1986a). Researchers have also had difficulty in identifying animal models for research that replicate the HIV disease mechanisms in humans.

Other issues involve the ethical considerations in using human subjects for clinical trials of the vaccine. Clinical trials of an HIV vaccine will require the following three phases:

1. Phase 1 will be conducted on healthy adult volunteers who are not practicing high-risk behaviors to determine if the vaccine is safe and has no adverse effects.
2. Phase 2 will utilize high-risk volunteers to ascertain optimum vaccine dosage for safety and effective immunization response.
3. Phase 3 will be double-blind, randomized trials using high-

risk subjects to determine if the immunized and nonim-
munized groups differ in AIDS incidence.

In examining the research involved in developing the vaccine,
many ethical questions arise. How will vaccine-induced seroconversion, that is, becoming antibody positive as a result of vaccination, affect a subject's emotional health and social welfare?
Will this be a deterrent to recruiting subjects for the clinical trials?
How will volunteers for these vaccine studies be obtained?

Liability issues are also of great concern and may slow the
development, production, and distribution of a vaccine. Over
the past several years, pharmaceutical companies have with-
drawn from production of vaccines because of liability issues. To
overcome these barriers, the state of California recently enacted
legislation to protect any manufacturer of an FDA-approved
AIDS vaccine distributed in California from liability as a result of
product defects or warnings. Although the legislation also provides a vaccine compensation fund for those persons injured by
the vaccine, no compensation provisions were included for
those injured as a result of clinical trials (Koff & Hoth, 1988).

Hopefully, an intense research effort underwritten by the federal government, universities, pharmaceutical companies, and
the private sector will result in an efficacious vaccine within the
next decade.

DISTRIBUTING CONDOMS AND STERILE NEEDLES

In an effort to curb the spread of AIDS, health and social
service agencies throughout this country are proposing projects
to distribute condoms and sterile needles. Much controversy has
surfaced about these proposals, including concerns that we are
encouraging IV drug use and sexual promiscuity. In essence,
these programs are attempting to reach populations who are
already engaged in high-risk behaviors and assist them in protecting themselves from AIDS. Logically speaking, getting these

groups to protect themselves with condoms and sterile needles will be easier than changing their sexual and drug behaviors.

Portland, Oregon, has announced the first program in the nation to distribute hypodermic needles to drug users. Funded by the American Foundation for AIDS Research, Outside-In will utilize the $67,000 grant to counsel 125 drug users and exchange used needles for sterile ones. This one-year project will study whether an intervention of this type can control the transmission of AIDS. Subjects will have periodic blood tests and results will be compared with a matched group of drug users from 11 other U.S. cities ("Portland Will Experiment", 1988). New York City and Boston also have plans for distribution of free sterile needles but are awaiting approval from lawmakers. In Europe, Holland has established needle exchanges. Research there does not demonstrate increased drug use as a result of the availability of sterile needles (DesJarlais & Friedman, 1988).

Distribution of condoms in universities and health departments has also been initiated in many locations. Recently, the state of Michigan included condoms in its Medicaid drug formulary. No prescriptions will be needed to obtain condoms, and men as well as women are eligible to receive them. To monitor dispensing of the condoms, only 24 condoms will be given to an individual at one time ("Condoms Under Medicaid," 1988). Finally, New York City has provided $1 million in funds for distributing condoms and literature to community organizations, family planning clinics, and sexually transmitted disease (STD) clinics (Joseph, 1988).

SUMMARY

As we have seen, every available prevention effort from AIDS education to distribution of condoms is now underway in this country. For the most part, AIDS prevention efforts represent a struggle to contain this dangerous disease as expeditiously as possible. All available preventive approaches must be mobilized. All organizations, companies, agencies, and institutions must be involved. Every man, woman, and child must be protected.

REFERENCES

Benza, J., & R. Zumwalde (1986) *Preventing AIDS: A Practical Guide for Everyone.* Cincinnati, Ohio: Jalsco, Inc.

Chin, J. (1988) Strategies for the prevention and control of AIDS: The California experience. In R. Schinazi & A. Nahmias, eds., *AIDS in Children, Adolescents & Heterosexual Adults*, pp. 13–14. New York: Elsevier Publishing Co.

Christ, G., & L. Wiener (1985) Psychosocial issues in AIDS. In V. DeVita, S. Hellman & S. Rosenberg, eds., *AIDS: Etiology, Diagnosis, Treatment and Prevention*, pp. 275–297. Philadelphia: J. B. Lippincott Co.

Commission says public health response to AIDS seriously lacks funds and lacks coordination. (1988) *The Nation's Health* (August) p. 16.

Condoms under Medicaid (1988) *The Nation's Health* (August) p. 12.

DesJarlais, D., & S. Friedman (1988) AIDS prevention among IV drug users: Experience in high prevalence states. In R. Schinazi & A. Nahmias, eds., *AIDS in Children, Adolescents and Heterosexual Adults*, pp. 396–397. New York: Elsevier Publishing Co.

Eldridge, F. (1988) Legal aspects related to possible measures for the prevention of perinatal human immunodeficiency virus infection. In R. Schinazi & A. Nahmias, eds., *AIDS in Children, Adolescents and Heterosexual Adults*, pp. 210–211. New York: Elsevier Publishing Co.

Hearst, N., & S. Hulley (1988) Preventing the heterosexual spread of AIDS. *Journal of the American Medical Association* 259(16):2428–2432.

Holland, N. (1987) Blood policy dynamics: An overview. In J. Griggs, S. Rogers, D. Gould & G. Schneider, eds., *AIDS*

Public Policy Dimensions, pp. 101–106. New York:
United Hospital Fund of New York.

Institute of Medicine, National Academy of Sciences (1986b)
*Confronting AIDS: Directions for Public Health, Health
Care and Research.* Washington, D.C.: National Academy Press.

Institute of Medicine, National Academy of Sciences (1986a)
Mobilizing against AIDS. Cambridge, Massachusetts:
Harvard University Press.

Joseph, S. (1988) AIDS in New York City: Public health challenges. In R. Schinazi & A. Nahmias, eds., *AIDS in
Children, Adolescents and Heterosexual Adults.* New
York: Elsevier Publishing Co.

Kibrick, S. (1988) The adolescent and education: Introductory
remarks. In R. Schinazi & A. Nahmias, eds., *AIDS in
Children, Adolescents and Heterosexual Adults,* pp.
323–324. New York: Elsevier Publishing Co.

Koff, W., & D. Hoth (1988) Development and testing of AIDS
vaccines. *Science* 241:426–432.

MacDonald, D. (1986) Public health plan for prevention and
control of AIDS and the AIDS virus. *Public Health
Reports* 101:341–348.

New York medical societies sue for AIDS contact tracing
(1988) *The Nation's Health* (August).p. 8.

Next to abstinence, condoms are best way to prevent AIDS
(1988) in *Common Sense about AIDS* (Available from
American Health Consultants, Inc., 67 Peachtree Park
Drive NE, Atlanta, GA 30309–1397).

Pindyck, J. (1987) AIDS and the blood service system. In J.
Griggs, S. Rogers, D. Gould & G. Schneider, eds., *AIDS
Public Policy Dimensions,* pp. 85–100. New York:
United Hospital Fund of New York.

Portland will experiment with needle exchange for addicts
(1988) *The Nation's Health* (August) p. 8.

Reagan seeks new AIDS policies after report (1988) *The
Nation's Health* (August) p. 5.

Stein, J. (1987) Employers' role in preventing disease. *Business and Health* 4(4):46–48.

Wolfsy, C. (1988) AIDS and prostitution. In R. Schinazi & A. Nahmias, eds., *AIDS in Children, Adolescents and Heterosexual Adults*, pp. 168–169. New York: Elsevier Publishing Co.

APPENDIX A

HUMAN IMMUNODEFICIENCY VIRUS (HIV) INFECTION CLASSIFICATION

BACKGROUND

The increasing importance of HIV infection has created a demand for more specific disease codes that would allow public health officials, clinical researchers, and agencies that finance medical care to accurately monitor diagnoses of AIDS and other manifestations of HIV infection as they are coded on death certificates and medical records. Since the next revision of the ICD (ICD-10) will not become available for another 5 or 6 years, new codes for this infection were developed jointly by the Center for Infectious Diseases and the National Center for Health Statistics of the Centers for Disease Control.

When an interim classification was issued on October 1, 1986, it was anticipated that periodic revisions would be required. One such revision is the recent change in terminology characterizing the causative agent. In a memorandum dated April 17, 1987, the Assistant Secretary for Health recommended that the term "human immunodeficiency virus (HIV)" be used to identify the AIDS virus.

DEFINITIONS

This classification is not intended for purposes of staging or specifying severity of illness. Rather, it is based on well-defined groupings of disease manifestations most compatible with the manner in which patients with HIV infection are currently categorized by providers of

Effective January 1, 1988, *Morbidity and Mortality Weekly Report* 1987, 36 (no. S-7):1–24.

health-care services, clinical investigators, researchers, and public health officials. Thus, the spectrum of HIV infection is divided into three categories:

1. HIV infection with specified secondary infections or malignant neoplasms, or AIDS (042).
2. HIV infection with other specified manifestations in the absence of either specified secondary infections or malignant neoplasms (043).
3. Other HIV infection not classifiable above (044).

TERMINOLOGY

The use of unacceptable terminology and abbreviations should be discouraged. Acquired immunodeficiency syndrome (AIDS) is not synonymous with HIV infection or with such terms as pre-AIDS and AIDS-related complex or syndromes.

Any record that reports "possible," "probable," or "questionable" AIDS, not confirmed, without manifestations listed should be returned to the physician for clarification.

HOW TO USE THIS CLASSIFICATION

To use these codes correctly, the physician must provide complete information and state the relationship between HIV infection and other conditions. It will not be unusual for a patient suffering from HIV infection to be admitted for an unrelated condition.

The classification requires that the relationship between the HIV infection, the manifestations, and other listed conditions be identified. The term "with" implies that the condition or manifestation of HIV infection need only be listed on the record. Terms such as "and" and "in association with" will be considered in the same manner as "with."

The term "due to" is used in this classification to denote a causal relationship. The broad definition of "due to" is implied here as it is used in the International Classification of Diseases, 9th Revision.

> The words "due to (or as a consequence of)" which appear
> on the form of medical certificate include not only etiol-
> ogical or pathological sequences, but also sequences

where there is no such direct causation but where an antecedent condition is believed to have prepared the way for the direct cause by damage to tissues or impairment of function even after a long interval (World Health Organization, 1977, p. 700).

All manifestations of HIV infection must be coded. The alphabetical table will help the coder select the most appropriate code for the HIV infection in association with the most common manifestations. Other manifestations not found on the table may be reported; the selection of the appropriate 042–044 code is determined solely by the terminology used for the HIV infection. Codes 042, 043, and 044 are mutually exclusive and should never be listed together on the same record. Priority is given to 042 over 043 and 044; 043 is given priority over 044.

Only *one* code from the 042–044 series should be used. For instance, a patient with candidiasis of the lung (112.4), Kaposi's sarcoma (173), and HIV infection described as AIDS would be assigned only one 042 code. The coder should select a single HIV code based on a discussion with the attending physician as to the most descriptive code for the admission. This code may change during subsequent admissions.

In morbidity use, selection of the principal diagnosis should be based on the information contained in the individual medical record of the patient's hospitalization. Selection of the principal diagnosis and a secondary diagnosis applies only to hospitalized patients. The HIV infection codes can be used as either the principal or a secondary diagnosis. The notes "with" and "due to HIV infection" do not imply sequencing.

This classification system will be used while additional scientific information on the pathogenesis and natural history of HIV infection accumulates. This revision follows 1 year of use. This system will continue to be reviewed for its appropriateness in classifying HIV infection and its disease manifestations.

HUMAN IMMUNODEFICIENCY VIRUS (HIV) INFECTION (042–044)

Note: In this classification, the following terms are used to define and to represent other terms that are referable to these categories 042–044.

1. AIDS
    Acquired immune deficiency syndrome
    Acquired immunodeficiency syndrome
2. AIDS-like syndrome:
    AIDS-like disease (illness) (syndrome)
    AIDS-related complex
    AIDS-related conditions
    ARC
    Pre-AIDS
    Prodromal AIDS
3. HIV infection (disease) (illness)
    AAV(disease) (illness) (infection)
    AIDS-associated retrovirus (disease) (illness) (infection)
    AIDS-related virus (disease) (illness) (infection)
    AIDS virus (disease) (illness) (infection)
    ARV (disease) (illness) (infection)
    Human immunodeficiency virus (disease) (illness) (infection)
    Human immunovirus (disease) (illness) (infection)
    Human T-cell lymphotropic virus-III (disease) (illness) (infection)
    HTLV-III (disease) (illness) (infection)
    HTLV-III/LAV (disease) (illness) (infection)
    LAV (disease) (illness) (infection)
    LAV/HTLV-III (disease) (illness) (infection)
    Lymphadenopathy-associated virus (disease) (illness) (infection)

042 Human immunodeficiency virus infection with specified conditions. Includes: Acquired immunodeficiency syndrome (AIDS)

042.0 With specified infections (With HIV infection)
    Includes only:
        candidiasis of lung (112.4)
        coccidiosis (007.2)
          cryptosporidiosis (007.2)
          isosporiasis (007.2)
        cryptococcosis (117.5)
        pneumocystosis (136.3)
        progressive multifocal leukoencephalopathy (046.3)
        toxoplasmosis (130)

042.1 Causing other specified infections
    Includes only these diseases due to HIV infection:
      candidiasis
        disseminated (112.5)
        of mouth: (112.0)
          skin and nails (112.3)
          other and unspecified sites (112.8, 112.9)
          (excludes: 112.1, 112.2, 112.4)
      coccidioidomycosis (114)
      cytomegalic inclusion disease (078.5)
      herpes simplex (054)
      herpes zoster (053)
      histoplasmosis (115)
      mycobacteriosis, other and unspecified
        (031.8, 031.9) (Excludes: 031.0,031.1)
      Nocardia infection (039)
      opportunistic mycoses (118)
      pneumonia:
        NOS (486)
        viral NOS (480.9)
      Salmonella infections (003.1-003.9)
        (excludes: gastroenteritis 003.0)
      septicemia (038)
      strongyloidiasis (127.2)
      tuberculosis (010–018)

042.2 With specified malignant neoplasms
    Includes only: With HIV infection
      Burkitt's tumor or lymphoma (200.2)
      Kaposi's sarcoma (173)
      immunoblastic sarcoma (200.8)
      primary lymphoma of the brain (202.8)
      reticulosarcoma (200.0)

042.9 Acquired immunodeficiency syndrome, unspecified
    AIDS with other conditions classifiable elsewhere except as in
    042.0–042.2

043 Human immunodeficiency virus infection causing other specified conditions
    Includes: AIDS-like syndrome
                AIDS-related complex
                ARC
    Excludes: HIV infection classifiable to 042

043.0 Causing lymphadenopathy due to HIV infection
    Enlarged lymph nodes (785.6)
    Swollen glands (785.6)

043.1 Causing specified diseases of the central nervous system due to HIV infection
    Includes only:
        central nervous system:
            demyelinating disease NOS (341.9)
            disorders NOS (348.9, 349.9)
            non-arthropod-borne viral diseases,
            other and unspecified (049.8, 049.9)
            slow virus infection, other and
            unspecified (046.8, 046.9)
        dementia:
            NOS (298.9)
            organic (294.9)
            presenile (290.1)
        encephalitis (323.9)
        encephalomyelitis (348.9)
        encephalopathy (348.3)
        myelitis (323.9)
        myelopathy (336.9)
        organic brain syndrome NOS (nonpsychotic)
            (310.9) psychotic (294.9)

043.2 Causing other disorders involving the immune mechanism

043.3 Causing other specified conditions due to HIV infection
    Includes only:
        abnormal weight loss (783.2)
        abnormality, respiratory (786.0)
        agranulocytosis (288.0)

anemia:
  NOS (285.9)
  aplastic, other and unspecified (284.3, 284.9)
  deficiency (280–281)
  hemolytic, acquired (283)
arthritis:
  pyogenic (711.0)
  infective (711.9)
blindness or low vision (369)
blood and blood-forming organs, unspecified disease (289.9)
cachexia (799.4)
dermatomycosis (111)
dermatophytosis (110)
diarrhea (noninfectious) (558)
  infectious (009)
disease or disorder NOS:
  blood and blood-forming organs (289.9)
  salivary gland (527.9)
  skin and subcutaneous tissue (709.9)
dyspnea (786.0)
fatigue (780.7)
fever (780.6)
gastroenteritis (noninfectious) (558)
  infectious (009)
hepatomegaly (789.1)
hyperhidrosis (780.8)
hypersplenism (289.4)
infection: intestinal, ill-defined (009)
lack of expected physiological development in infant (783.4)
leukoplakia of oral mucosa (tongue) (528.6)
malabsorption, intestinal (579.9)
malaise (780.7)
neuralgia NOS (729.2)
neuritis NOS (729.2)
nutritional deficiencies (260-269)
pneumonitis, lymphoid, interstitial (516.8)
polyneuropath (357.0, 357.8, 357.9)
pyrexia (780.6)
radiculitis NOS (729.2)
rash NOS (782.1)

retinal vascular changes (362.1)
retinopathy, background (362.1)
splenomegaly (789.2)
thrombocytopenia, secondary and unspecified (287.4, 287.5)
volume depletion (276.5)

*043.9 Acquired immunodeficiency syndrome-related complex, un-
specified*
AIDS-related complex (ARC) with other conditions classifiable
elsewhere except as in 042.0–043.3

044 Other human immunodeficiency virus infection
Excludes: HIV infection classifiable to 042–043

044.0 Causing specified acute infections due to HIV infection
Includes only:
acute lymphadenitis (683)
aseptic meningitis (047.9)
viral infection ("infectious mononucleosis-like
syndrome") (079.9)

044.9 Human immunodeficiency virus infection, unspecified
HIV infection with other conditions classifiable
elsewhere except as in 042.0–044.0

*795.8 Positive serological or viral culture findings for human immu-
nodeficiency virus (HIV)*

REFERENCES

World Health Organization (1977) *Manual of the International Statistical Classification of Diseases, Injuries, and Causes of Death,
Based on the Recommendation of the Ninth Revision Conference, 1975.* Geneva: World Health Organization.

APPENDIX B

U.S. OFFICE OF PERSONNEL MANAGEMENT POLICY: ACQUIRED IMMUNE DEFICIENCY SYNDROME (AIDS) IN THE WORKPLACE

INTRODUCTION

This information and guidance is designed to assist Federal agencies in establishing effective AIDS education programs and in fairly and effectively handling AIDS-related personnel situations in the workplace. In this guidance, the term AIDS is used to refer either to the general AIDS phenomenon or to clinically diagnosed AIDS as a medical condition. HIV (human immunodeficiency virus) is used when the discussion is referring to the range of medical conditions which HIV-infected persons might have (i.e., immunological and/or neurological impairment in early HIV infection to clinically diagnosed AIDS).

GENERAL POLICY

Guidelines issued by the Public Health Service's Centers for Disease Control (CDC) dealing with AIDS in the workplace state that "the kind of nonsexual person-to-person contact that generally occurs among workers and clients or consumers in the workplace does not pose a risk for transmission of [AIDS]." Therefore, HIV-infected employees should be allowed to continue working as long as they are able to maintain acceptable performance and do not pose a safety or health threat to themselves or others in the workplace. If performance or safety problems arise, agencies are encouraged to address them by applying existing Federal and agency personnel policies and practices. (See also Public Health Service's guidelines for health-care workers.)

HIV infection can result in medical conditions which impair the employee's health and ability to perform safely and effectively. In these cases, agencies should treat HIV-infected employees in the same manner as employees who suffer from other serious illnesses. This means, for example, that employees may be granted sick leave or leave without pay when they are incapable of performing their duties or when they have medical appointments. In this regard, agencies are encouraged to consider accommodation of employees' AIDS-related conditions in the same manner as they would other medical conditions which warrant such consideration.

Also, there is no medical basis for employees refusing to work with such fellow employees or agency clients who are HIV infected. Nevertheless, the concerns of these employees should be taken seriously and should be addressed with appropriate information and counseling. In addition, employees, such as health-care personnel, who may come into direct contact with the body fluids of persons having the AIDS virus, should be provided appropriate information and equipment to minimize the risks of such contact.

OPM encourages agencies to consider the following guidelines when establishing AIDS education programs and in carrying out their personnel management responsibilities.

I. AIDS INFORMATION AND EDUCATION PROGRAMS

There are several important considerations in establishing effective AIDS information and education programs. The following guidance is intended to help agencies develop methods for establishing successful programs.

A. Timing and Scope of AIDS Information and Education Efforts

AIDS information and education programs are most effective if they begin before a problem situation arises relative to AIDS and employee concerns. Experience in the private sector has demonstrated that employees' level of receptivity to accurate information will be higher when management has a policy of open communications and when educational efforts are initiated before a problem situation occurs. Education and information should be of an ongoing nature. This approach will reassure employees of management's commitment to open communications and employees will receive updated information about AIDS. By providing AIDS information to all employees, agencies will enhance employees' understanding about the nature and transmission of the disease.

B. Educational Vehicles

Education and information efforts may be carried out in a variety of ways. Agency news bulletins, personnel management directives, meetings with employees, expert speakers and counselors, question-and-answer sessions, films and videotapes, employee newsletters, union publications, factsheets, pamphlets, and brochures are likely to be effective means of providing information to employees about AIDS.

C. Employee Assistance Programs

For employees who have personal concerns about AIDS, agency employee assistance programs (EAPs) can be an excellent source of information and counseling, and can provide referrals, as requested, to community testing, treatment, and other resources. EAPs can also provide counseling to employees who have apprehensions regarding the communicability of the disease or other related concerns. Because EAPs are in a unique position to offer information and assistance, agencies are encouraged to establish AIDS information, counseling, and referral capabilities in their EAPs and to make employees and supervisors aware of available services. In addition, EAPs can be a good source of managerial/supervisory training on AIDS in the workplace. As with other services provided by the EAP, strict adherence to applicable privacy and confidentiality requirements must be observed when advising employees with AIDS-related concerns. In addition to services provided by the EAP, the agency's occupational health program, health unit, or medical staff should be prepared to assist employees seeking information and counseling on AIDS.

D. Training and Guidance for Managers and Supervisors

Supervisors and managers should be prepared to deal with employee concerns and other issues related to AIDS in the workplace. Agencies should consider, therefore, conducting ongoing training and education programs on AIDS for their managers and supervisors on the medical and personnel management dimensions of AIDS. These programs can be used to educate managers and supervisors on the latest research on AIDS in the workplace, to provide advice on how to recognize and handle situations which arise in their organizations, and to convey the importance of maintaining the confidentiality of any medical and other information about employees' health status. In addition, managers and supervisors should be given a point of contact within the agency where they can call to obtain further information or to discuss situations which arise in their work units. Agencies should attempt to initiate training and guidance activities before problems occur.

E. Sources of Information and Educational Materials

A great deal of information about AIDS is available to Federal agencies. OPM encourages agencies to explore various sources of information and to keep abreast of the latest research on AIDS in the workplace. The U.S. Public Health Service (PHS) has developed a great deal of material on the medical and other aspects of AIDS. Information about AIDS can be obtained requesting it from PHS offices or from the AIDS Clearinghouse (America Responds to AIDS, P.O. Box 6003, Rockville, MD 20850; telephone (800) 342-7514). PHS offices are located throughout the country and can be contacted for information relating to AIDS. (See section III for a listing of PHS regional office locations.) In addition, the American Red Cross has developed an extensive assortment of educational materials on AIDS. Information about the materials available through PHS and other sources is contained in section III.

II. PERSONNEL MANAGEMENT ISSUES AND CONSIDERATIONS

When AIDS becomes a matter of concern in the workplace, a variety of personnel issues may arise. Basically, these issues should be addressed within the framework of existing procedures, guidance, statutes, case law, and regulation. Following is a brief discussion of AIDS-related issues which could arise in various personnel management areas, along with some basic guidance on how to approach and resolve

such issues. Agencies are cautioned that, as with any complex personnel management matter, the resolution of a specific problem must be
based on a thorough assessment of that problem and how it is affected
by contemporary information and guidance about AIDS, current law
and regulation bearing on the involved issue, and the agency's own
policies and needs.

A. Employees' Ability to Work

An HIV-infected employee may develop a variety of medical conditions. These conditions can range all the way from immunological and/
or neurological impairment in early stages of HIV infection to clinically
diagnosed AIDS. At some point, a concern may arise whether such an
employee, given his or her medical condition, can perform the duties
of the position in a safe and reliable manner. This concern will typically
arise at a point when the HIV-infected employee suffers health problems which affect his or her ability to report for duty or perform. Also,
in some situations the concern may stem from the results of a medical
examination required by the employee's position. Under OPM's regulations in 5 C.F.R. Part 339, Medical Determination Related to Employability, it is primarily the employee's responsibility to produce medical
documentation regarding the extent to which a medical condition is
affecting availability for duty or job performance. However, when the
employee does not produce sufficient documentation to allow agency
management to make an informed decision about the extent of the
employee's capabilities, the agency may offer, and in some cases order,
the employee to undergo a medical examination. Accurate and timely
medical information will allow the agency to consider alternatives to
keeping the employee in his or her position if there are serious questions
about safe and reliable performance. It will also help determine whether
the HIV-infected employee's medical condition is sufficiently disabling
to entitle the employee to be considered for reasonable accommodation under the Rehabilitation Act of 1973 (29 U.S.C. S 794).

B. Privacy and Confidentiality

Because of the nature of the disease, HIV-infected employees will
have understandable concerns over confidentiality and privacy in

connection with medical documentation and other information relating to their condition. Agencies should be aware that any medical documentation submitted to an agency for the purpose of an employment decision and made part of the file pertaining to that decision becomes a "record" covered by the Privacy Act. The Privacy Act generally forbids agencies to disclose a record which the Act covers without the consent of the subject of the record. However, these records are available to agency officials who have a need to know the information for an appropriate management purpose. Officials who have access to such information are required to maintain the confidentiality of that information. In addition, supervisors, managers, and others included in making and implementing personnel management decisions involving employees with AIDS should strictly observe applicable privacy and confidentiality requirements.

C. Leave Administration

HIV-infected employees may request sick or annual leave or leave without pay to pursue medical care or to recuperate from the ill effects of his or her medical condition. In these situations the agency should make its determination on whether to grant leave in the same manner as it would for other employees with medical conditions.

D. Changes in Work Assignment

Agencies considering changes such as job restructuring, detail, reassignment, or flexible scheduling for HIV-infected employees should do so in the same manner as they would for other employees whose medical conditions affect the employee's ability to perform in a safe and reliable manner. In considering changes in work assignments, agencies should observe established policies governing qualification requirements, internal placement, and other staffing requirements.

E. Employee Conduct

There may be situations where fellow employees express reluctance or threaten refusal to work with HIV-infected employees. Such reluctance is often based on misinformation or lack of information about the transmission of HIV. There is, however, no known risk of transmission of HIV through normal workplace contacts, according to leading medical research. Nevertheless, OPM recognizes that the presence of such fears, if unaddressed in an appropriate and timely manner, can be disruptive to an organization. Usually an agency will be able to deal effectively with such situations through information, counseling, and other means. However, in situations where such measures do not solve the problem and where management determines that an employee's unwarranted threat or refusal to work with an HIV-infected employee is impeding or disrupting the organization's work, it should consider appropriate corrective or disciplinary action against the threatening or disruptive employee(s). In other situations, management may be faced with an HIV-infected employee who is having performance or conduct problems. Management should deal with these problems through appropriate counseling, remedial, and, if necessary, disciplinary measures. In pursuing appropriate action in these situations, management should be sensitive to the possible contribution of anxiety over the illness to work behavior and to the requirements of existing Federal and agency personnel policies, including any obligations the agency may have to consider reasonable accommodation of the HIV-infected employee.

F. Insurance

HIV-infected employees can continue their coverages under the Federal Employees Health Benefits (FEHB) Program and/or the Federal Employees' Group Life Insurance (FEGLI) Program in the same manner as other employees. Their continued participation in either or both of these programs would not be jeopardized solely because of their medical condition. The health benefits plans cannot exclude coverage for medically necessary health-care services based on an individual's health status or a pre-existing condition. Similarly, the death benefits payable under the FEGLI Program are not cancellable solely because of the individual's current health status. However, *any* employee who is in a leave-without-pay (LWOP) status for 12 continuous months faces the statutory loss of FEHB and FEGLI coverage but has the privilege of conversion to a private policy without having to undergo a physical examination. Employees who are seeking to cancel previous declina-

tions and/or obtain *additional* levels of FEGLI coverage must prove to
the satisfaction of the Office of Federal Employees' Group Life Insurance that they are in reasonably good heath. Any employee exhibiting
symptoms of any serious and life-threatening illness would necessarily
be denied the request for additional coverage.

G. Disability Retirement

HIV-infected employees may be eligible for disability retirement if
their medical condition warrants and if they have the requisite years of
Federal service to qualify. OPM considers applications for disability
retirement from employees with AIDS in the same mannner as for other
employees, focusing on the extent of the employee's incapacitation and
ability to perform his or her assigned duties. OPM makes every effort to
expedite any applications where the employee's illness is in an advanced stage and is life threatening.

H. Labor-Management Relations

AIDS in the workplace may be an appropriate area for cooperative
labor-management activities, particularly with respect to providing
employees education and information and alleviating AIDS-related
problems that may emerge in the workplace. In addition, to the extent
that an agency proposed AIDS-related policies or programs which
would affect the working conditions of bargaining-unit employees,
unions must be accorded any rights they may have to bargain or be
consulted as provided for under 5 U.S.C. Chapter 71.

I. Health and Safety Standards

In 1985, the CDC published guidelines relating to the prevention of
HIV transmission in most workplace settings, *CDC Recommendations
for Preventing Transmission of Infection with HIV in the Workplace*, 34
MMWR 681 (November 15, 1985). The CDC published specialized
guidelines in 1987 relating to health-care workers (which in part
updated the health-care worker provisions contained in the workplace
guidelines), *CDC Recommendations for Prevention of HIV Transmis-*

sion in Health-Care Settings, 36 MMWR Supp. no. 2S (August 21, 1987). The Department of Health and Human Services (HHS) and the Occupational Safety and Health Administration (OSHA) of the Department of Labor have initiated a program to ensure compliance with safety and health guidelines and standards designed to protect health-care workers from blood-borne diseases, including AIDS. See Department of Labor/Department of Health and Human Services — Joint Advisory Notice: *Protection Against Occupational Exposure to Hepatitis B Virus (HBV) and Human Immunodeficiency Virus (HIV)*, 52 Fed. Reg. 41818 (October 30, 1987). The CDC and OSHA/HHS guidance is intended to increase the availability and use of educational information and personal protective equipment and to improve workplace practices bearing on the transmission of AIDS and other bloodborne disease. OPM strongly encourages agencies, especially those with employees occupying health-care and related positions, to establish health and safety practices consistent with this guidance. Sources are available in OSHA to discuss the published guidelines.

J. Blood Donations

One area of personnel management which agencies may overlook when considering AIDS policies and practices is employee blood donations. OPM joins the American Red Cross in urging agencies to encourage employees to consider donating blood. Under guidelines established by the American Red Cross, there is no risk of contracting AIDS from giving blood. However, fears associated with AIDS have contributed to a situation where many of the nation's blood banks are in short supply. This situation threatens the health status of the American public.

As part of its effort to educate the public so as to overcome these fears, the American Red Cross has produced three publications which address blood donations where AIDS is an issue. These publications are: "You Can't Get AIDS From Giving Blood, But Fear Can Run Us Dry," "What You Must Know Before Giving Blood," and "AIDS and the Safety of the Nation's Blood Supply." These publications are available through your local Red Cross chapter or by contacting the Red Cross National Headquarters AIDS Public Education Program (by writing to 1730 "D" Street, NW, Washington, DC 20006 or by calling (202) 639-3223).

III. AIDS INFORMATION SOURCES

A. Federal Government Resources

1. *Department of Health and Human Services*
U. S. Public Health Service
Hubert H. Humphrey Building
200 Independence Avenue, SW
Washington, DC 20201

Lead agency in the distribution of AIDS information, both general and technical in nature. The following materials have been prepared by the Public Health Service and are available to the public free of charge through the National AIDS Clearinghouse (address listed below).

Surgeon General's Report on Acquired Immune Deficiency Syndrome (English and Spanish)

What You Should Know About AIDS

Facts About AIDS

Coping with AIDS

Joint Advisory Notice: Department of Labor/Department of Health and Human Services — Protection Against Occupational Exposure to Hepatitis B Virus (HBV) and Human Immunodeficiency Virus (HIV) (for health-care workers and their employers)

Pamphlet series published in cooperation with the American Red Cross:

- AIDS, Sex, and You
- If Your Test for Antibody to the AIDS Virus is Positive
- Facts About AIDS and Drug Abuse
- Gay and Bisexual Men and AIDS
- AIDS and the Safety of the Nation's Blood Supply
- Caring for the AIDS Patient at Home
- AIDS and Your Job — Are There Risks?
- AIDS and Children: Information for Teachers and School Officials
- AIDS and Children: Information for Parents of School-Age Children

AIDS Update (a periodic news bulletin)

Morbidity and Mortality Weekly Report (Available from the Superintendent of Documents)

How to Order Publications   All the publications listed above except the "AIDS Update" and the *Morbidity and Mortality Weekly Report* can be ordered by calling the Public Health Service's National AIDS Hotline (1-800-342-AIDS) or by writing to:

National AIDS Clearinghouse
P. O. Box 6003
Rockville, MD 20850

The "AIDS Update" can be ordered by calling (202) 245-6867 or by writing to the address below.

Office of Public Affairs
Public Health Service
Room 725-H
200 Independence Avenue, SW
Washington, DC 20201

The *Morbidity and Mortality Weekly Report* is prepared by the Centers for Disease Control, Atlanta, Georgia, and is available on a paid subscription basis from the Superintendent of Documents by calling (202) 783-3238 or by writing to the address below.

Superintendent of Documents
U. S. Government Printing Office
Washington, DC 20402

The Public Health Service also operates an AIDS Hotline toll-free (800) 342-AIDS. A recorded message provides general information to callers concerning AIDS. Also provides a toll-free number for answers to specific questions about AIDS and information about nationwide AIDS-antibody testing sites.

Public Health Service Regional Health Administrators   The following is a listing of the addresses and telephone numbers of the Public Health Service Regional Health Administrators:

Region I
Connecticut, Maine, Massachusetts, New Hampshire, Rhode Island,
Vermont

John F. Kennedy Federal Building
Room 1400
Boston, MA 02203
(617) 565-1426 (FTS) 835-1426

Region II
New Jersey, New York, Puerto Rico, Virgin Islands

26 Federal Plaza, Room 3337
New York, NY 10278
(212/FTS) 264-2560

Region III
Delaware, District of Columbia, Maryland, Pennsylvania, Virginia,
West Virginia

Gateway Building #1
3535 Market Street
Mailing Address: P. O. Box 13716
Philadelphia, PA 19101
(215/FTS) 596-6637

Region IV
Alabama, Florida, Georgia, Kentucky, Mississippi, North Carolina,
South Carolina, Tennessee

101 Marietta Tower, Suite 1106
Atlanta, GA 30323
(404) 331-2316 (FTS) 242-2316

Region V
Illinois, Indiana, Michigan, Minnesota, Ohio, Wisconsin

300 South Wacker Drive, 34th Floor
Chicago, IL 60606
(312/FTS) 353-1385

Region VI
Arkansas, Louisiana, New Mexico, Oklahoma, Texas

1200 Main Tower Building
Room 1800
Dallas, TX 75202
(214) 767-3879 (FTS) 729-3879

Region VII
Iowa, Kansas, Missouri, Nebraska

601 East 12th Street, 5th Floor
Kansas City, MO 64106
(816)426-3291 (FTS) 867-3291

Region VIII
Colorado, Montana, North Dakota, South Dakota, Utah, Wyoming

1961 Stout Street
Denver, CO 80294
(303) 844-6163 (FTS) 564-6163

Region IX
American Samoa, Arizona, California, Guam, Hawaii, Nevada, Trust
Territory of the Pacific Islands, Commonwealth of Northern Mariana
Islands

50 United Nations Plaza, Room 327
San Francisco, CA 94102
(415/FTS) 556-5810

Region X
Alaska, Idaho, Oregon, Washington

2901 Third Avenue, M. S. 402
Seattle, WA 98121
(206) 442-0430 (FTS) 399-0430

2. Department of Labor

Establishes and enforces health and safety standards in the health care workplace. Trains health and safety inspectors in applying OSHA guidelines.

Occupational Safety and Health Administration
Room South 2316
200 Constitution Avenue, NW
Washington, DC 20210

3. U. S. Office of Personnel Management

Establishes personnel management policies for the Federal Sector. Administers the Federal employee pay, retirement, and benefits programs. Provides technical assistance and support to agencies in administering their personnel programs.

Personnel Systems and Oversight Group
Office of Employee and Labor Relations
Office of Personnel Management
1900 E street, NW
Room 7635
Washington, DC 20415
(202) 653-8551

B. AIDS Prevention Program Project Directors and Coordinators

The U.S. Public Health Service recommends the use of state and local health agencies for additional information. Area testing sites and information concerning state health policies and services available to individuals with AIDS can be obtained from local health offices. For convenience, below is a list of AIDS Prevention Program Project Directors and Coordinators compiled by the Centers for Disease Control in Atlanta.

ALABAMA

Department of Public Health
State Office Building
Room 252
501 Dexter Avenue
Montgomery, AL 36130
(205) 261-5017

ALASKA

State Epidemiologist
Division of Public Health
P.O. Box 240249
Anchorage, AK 99524-0249
(907) 561-4406

ARIZONA

Division of Disease Prevention
Office of Infectious Disease
3008 N. Third Street
Room 103
Pheniz, AZ 85012
(602) 230-5819

ARKANSAS

Department of Health
AIDS Prevention Program
4815 West Markham
Room 455
Little Rock, AR 72205-3867
(501) 661-2140

CALIFORNIA

Office of AIDS
California Department of
    Health
1812 14th Street

Room 200
Sacramento, CA 95814
(916) 445-0553

AIDS Activity Office
Department of Public Health
101 Grove Street, Room 323
San Francisco, CA 94102
(415) 864-5571

Department of Health Services
AIDS Program Office
313 N. Figueroa Street
Room 1014
Los Angeles, CA 90012
(213) 974-7803

COLORADO

Department of Health
STD Control Program
4210 East 11th Avenue
Denver, CO 80220
(303) 398-0855
(FTS) 564-0855

CONNECTICUT

AIDS Program Coordinator
Department of Health Services
150 Washington Street
Hartford, CT 06106
(203) 566-1157

DELAWARE

Health and Social Services
Division of Public Health
802 Silver Lake Boulevard
Dover, DE 19901
(302) 736-5617

DISTRICT OF COLUMBIA

Chief
Office of AIDS Activity
1875 Connecticut Avenue, NW
Washington, DC 20009
(202) 673-7700

FLORIDA

Health and Rehabilitation
    Services
1317 Winewood Boulevard
Tallahassee, FL 32303
(904) 487-2478

GEORGIA

Department of Human
    Resources
Community Health Section
878 Peachtree Street, NE,
Room 102
Atlanta, GA 30309
(404) 894-6428

GUAM

Department of Public Health
P.O. Box 2816
Agana, Guam 96910
(671) 734-2964

HAWAII

Department of Health
STD Control Program
1250 Punchbowl Street
Honolulu, HI 96813
(808) 548-4580

IDAHO

Department of Health and
    Welfare
Bureau of Preventive
    Medicine
450 West State Street
Boise, ID 83720
(208) 334-4305

ILLINOIS

Director, AIDS Section
Department of Public Health
100 West Randolph
Suite 6-600
Chicago, IL 60602
(312) 917-4846

AIDS Project Director
Chicago Board of Health
50 West Washington
Room 233
Chicago, IL 60602
(312) 744-4358

INDIANA

State Board of Health
1330 West Michigan Street
Indianapolis, IN 46206-1964
(317) 633-8520

IOWA

Department of Health
Division of Disease
    Prevention
Lucas State Office Building
Des Moines, IA 50319
(515) 281-6438

KANSAS

Kansas Department of Health
Department of Health
   and Environment
Forbes Field
Topeka, KS 66620
(913) 296-5595

KENTUCKY

Kentucky AIDS Project
Department of Health Services
275 East Main Street
Frankfort, KY 40621
(502) 564-4804

LOUISIANA

Health and Human Resources
VD Control Section
P.O. Box 60630
New Orleans, LA 70160
(504) 568-5275
(FTS) 682-3948

MAINE

Department of Human Services
State House Station
Augusta, ME 04330
(207) 289-3747

MARYLAND

AIDS Administration
Health and Mental Hygiene
201 West Preston Street
Baltimore, MD 21201
(301) 225-6707

MASSACHUSETTS

State Laboratory Institute
Department of Public Health
305 South Street
Jamaica Plains, MA 02130
(617) 522-3700

MICHIGAN

Special Office on AIDS
Center for Health Promotion
P. O. Box 30035
Lansing, MI 48906
(517) 335-8399

MINNESOTA

Acute Disease Epi Section
Department of Health
717 SE Delaware Street
Minneapolis, MN 55440
(612) 632-5414

MISSISSIPPI

Department of Health
AIDS Program
P.O. Box 1700
Jackson, MS 39215-1700
(601) 960-7726
(FTS) 490-4491

MISSOURI

Divison of Health
AIDS Program
P.O. Box 570
Jefferson City, MO 65102-0570
(314) 751-6141

MONTANA

Department of Health
Health Education
Cogswell Building
Helena, MT 59620
(406) 444-4740

NEBRASKA

Department of Health
AIDS Program
301 Centennial Mall South
Lincoln, NE 68509
(402) 471-2937
(FTS) 541-2937

NEVADA

Division of Health
STD Control
505 E. King Street, Room 200
Carson City, NV 89710
(702) 885-4800

NEW HAMPSHIRE

Division of Public Health
  Services
Bureau of Disease Control
6 Hazen Drive
Concord, NH 03301
(603) 271-4477

NEW JERSEY

Department of Health
AIDS Program
CN 369, John Fetch Plaza
Trenton, NJ 08625
(609) 588-3520

NEW MEXICO

Health and Environment
AIDS Prevention Program
P.O. Box 968
Santa Fe, NM 87504-0968
(505) 827-0006

NEW YORK

Department of Health
AIDS Program
125 Worth Street
New York, NY 10013
(212) 566-7103

Department of Health
1315 Empire State Plaza
Albany, NY 12237
(518) 474-1689

NORTH CAROLINA

Communicable Disease
  Control
State of North Carolina
P.O. Box 2091
Raleigh, NC 27702
(919) 733-3419

NORTH DAKOTA

Department of Health
State Capitol Building
Bismarck, ND 58505
(701) 224-2378

OHIO

Department of Health
Epidemiology Division

246 N. High Street, 8th Floor
Columbus, OH 43266-0588
(614) 466-0265

OKLAHOMA

Department of Health
AIDS Division
P.O. Box 53551
Oklahoma City, OK 73152
(405) 271-4636

OREGON

AIDS Coordinator
Department of Human
   Resources
1400 SW Fifth Avenue
Portland, OR 97201
(503) 229-5792

PENNSYLVANIA

AIDS Education Manager
Division of Health Promotion
P.O. Box 90
Harrisburg, PA 17108
(717) 787-5900

PUERTO RICO

STD Control Program
Call Box STD
Caparra Heights Station
San Juan, PR 00922
(809) 754-8118

RHODE ISLAND

Department of Health
Disease Control

75 Davis Street
Providence, RI 02908
(401) 277-2362

SOUTH CAROLINA

Health and Environmental
   Control
2600 Bull Street
Columbia, SC 29201
(803) 734-5482

SOUTH DAKOTA

Department of Health
Communicable Disease
523 East Capitol
Pierre, SD 57501
(605) 773-3357

TENNESSEE

AIDS Education Coordinator
Department of Health
100 9th Avenue, North
Nashville, TN 37219-5405
(615) 741-7387
(FTS) 852-5638

TEXAS

Texas Department of Health
Director, AIDS Division
1100 West 49th Street
Austin, TX 78756
(512) 458-7207

UTAH

Bureau of Epidemiology
Utah Department of Health

P.O. Box 16660
Salt Lake City, UT 84116-0660
(801) 538-6191

VERMONT

Department of Health
STD Control Section
P.O. Box 70
Burlington, VT 05401
(802) 863-7245

VIRGINIA

VD Control Section
109 Governor Street
Room 722
Richmond, VA 23219
(804) 786-6267
(FTS) 936-6267

VIRGIN ISLANDS

Department of Health
Charles Harwood Complex
Christiansted
St. Croix, VI 00820
(809) 773-1059

WASHINGTON

Division of Health
Communicable Disease
    Section
Mail Stop LP-13
Olympia, WA 98504
(206) 753-5810
(FTS) 434-9559

WEST VIRGINIA

Director
AIDS Program
1800 Washington Street, East
Charleston, WV 25305
(304) 348-5358

WISCONSIN

Wisconsin Department
    of Health
1 West Wilson Street
Madison, WI 53701-0309
(608) 267-9007

WYOMING

AIDS HE/RR Program
Preventive Medicine
Hathaway Building, 4th Floor
Cheyenne, WY 82002
(307) 777-7953

APPENDIX C

U.S. PUBLIC HEALTH SERVICE GUIDELINES FOR COUNSELING AND ANTIBODY TESTING TO PREVENT HIV INFECTION AND AIDS

These guidelines are the outgrowth of the 1986 recommendations published in the *MMWR* (CDC, 1986a); the report on the February 24–25, 1987, Conference on Counseling and Testing (CDC, 1987b); and a series of meetings with representatives from the Association of State and Territorial Health Officials, the Association of State and Territorial Public Health Laboratory Directors, the Council of State and Territorial Epidemiologists, the National Association of County Health Officials, the United States Conference of Local Health Officers, and the National Association of State Alcohol and Drug Abuse Directors.

Human immunodeficiency virus (HIV), the causative agent of acquired immunodeficiency syndrome (AIDS) and related clinical manifestations, has been shown to be spread by sexual contact; by parenteral exposure to blood (most often through intravenous [IV] drug abuse) and, rarely, by other exposures to blood; and from an infected woman to her fetus or infant.

Persons exposed to HIV usually develop detectable levels of antibody against the virus within 6–12 weeks of infection. The presence of antibody indicated current infection, though many infected persons may have minimal or no clinical evidence of disease for years. Counseling and testing persons who are infected or at risk for acquiring HIV infection is an important component of prevention strategy (CDC, 1986a). Most of the estimated 1.0 to 1.5 million infected persons in the United States are unaware that they are infected with HIV. The primary

---

Morbidity and Mortality Weekly Report, 1987, 36 (31):509–514.

public health purposes of counseling and testing are to help uninfected individuals initiate and sustain behavioral changes that reduce their risk of becoming infected and to assist infected individuals in avoiding infecting others.

Along with the potential personal, medical, and public health benefits of testing for HIV antibody, public health agencies must be concerned about actions that will discourage the use of counseling and testing facilities, most notably the unauthorized disclosure of personal information and the possibility of inappropriate discrimination.

Priorities for public health counseling and testing should be based upon providing ready access to persons who are most likely to be infected or who practice high-risk behaviors, thereby helping to reduce further spread of infection. There are other considerations for determining testing priorities, including the likely effectiveness of preventing the spread of infection among persons who would not otherwise realize that they are at risk. Knowledge of the prevalence of HIV infection in different populations is useful in determining the most efficient and effective locations providing such services. For example, programs that offer counseling and testing to homosexual men, IV drug abusers, persons with hemophilia, sexual and/or needle-sharing partners of these persons, and patients of sexually transmitted disease clinics may be most effective since persons in these groups are at high risk for infection. After counseling and testing are effectively implemented in settings of high and moderate prevalence, consideration should be given to establishing programs in settings of lower prevalence.

INTERPRETATION OF HIV-ANTIBODY TEST RESULTS

A test for HIV antibody is considered positive when a sequence of tests, starting with a repeatedly reactive enzyme immunoassay (EIA) and including an additional, more specific assay, such as a Western blot, are consistently reactive.

The *sensitivity* of the currently licensed EIA tests is 99% or greater when performed under optimal laboratory conditions. Given this performance, the probability of a false-negative test result is remote, except during the first weeks after infection, before antibody is detectable.

The *specificity* of the currently licensed EIA tests is approximately 99% when repeatedly reactive tests are considered. Repeat testing of specimens initially reactive by EIA is required to reduce the likelihood of false-positive test results due to laboratory error. To further increase the specificity of the testing process, laboratories must use a supplemental test—most often the Western blot test—to validate repeatedly reactive EIA results. The sensitivity of the licensed Western blot test is comparable to that of the EIA, and it is highly specific when strict criteria are used for interpretation. Under ideal circumstances, the probability that a testing sequence will be falsely positive in a population with a low rate of infection ranges from less than 1 in 100,000 (Minnesota Department of Health, unpublished data) to an estimated 5 in 100,000 (Burke et al., 1987; Meyer & Pauker, 1987). Laboratories using different Western blot reagents or other tests or using less stringent interpretive criteria may experience higher rates of false-positive results.

Laboratories should carefully guard against human errors, which are likely to be the most common source of false-positive test results. All laboratories should anticipate the need for assuring quality performance of tests for HIV antibody by training personnel, establishing quality controls, and participating in performance evaluation systems. Health department laboratories should facilitate the quality assurance of the performance of laboratories in their jurisdiction.

GUIDELINES FOR COUNSELING AND TESTING FOR HIV ANTIBODY

These guidelines are based on public health considerations for HIV testing, including the principles of counseling before and after testing, confidentiality of personal information, and the understanding that a person may decline to be tested without being denied health care or other services, except where testing is required by law (Bayer, Levine, & Wolfe, 1986). Counseling before testing may not be practical when screening for HIV antibody is required. This is true for donors of blood, organs, and tissue; prisoners; and immigrants for whom testing is a Federal requirement as well as for persons admitted to state correctional institutions in states that require testing. When there is no counseling before testing, persons should be informed that testing for HIV antibody will be performed, that individual results will be kept confidential to the extent permitted by law, and that appropriate counseling will be offered. Individual counseling of those who are either HIV-antibody positive or at continuing risk for HIV infection is critical for reducing further

transmission and for ensuring timely medical care.
Specific recommendations follow:

1. **Persons who may have sexually transmitted disease.** All persons
   seeking treatment for a sexually transmitted disease, in all health-
   care settings including the offices of private physicians, should be
   routinely counseled and tested for HIV antibody. Except where
   counseling is required by law, individuals have the right to decline
   to be tested without being denied health care or other services.

2. **IV drug abusers.** All persons seeking treatment for IV drug abuse
   or having a history of IV drug abuse should be routinely counseled
   and tested for HIV antibody. Medical professionals in all health-
   care settings, including prison clinics, should seek a history of IV
   drug abuse from patients and should be aware of its implication for
   HIV infection. In addition, state and local health policy makers
   should address the following issues:

   • Treatment programs for IV drug abusers should be sufficiently
     available to allow persons seeking assistance to enter promptly
     and be encouraged to alter the behavior that places them and
     others at risk for HIV infection.
   • Outreach programs for IV drug abusers should be undertaken to
     increase their knowledge of AIDS and of ways to prevent HIV
     infection, to encourage them to obtain counseling and testing for
     HIV antibody, and to persuade them to be treated for substance
     abuse.

3. **Persons who consider themselves at risk.** All persons who consider themselves at risk for HIV infection should be counseled and
   offered testing for HIV antibody.

4. **Women of childbearing age.** All women of childbearing age with
   identifiable risks for HIV infection should be routinely counseled
   and tested for HIV antibody, regardless of the health-care setting.
   Each encounter between a health-care provider and a woman at
   risk and/or her sexual partners is an opportunity to reach them with
   information and education about AIDS and prevention of HIV
   infection. Women are at risk for HIV infection if they:

- Have used IV drugs
- Have engaged in prostitution
- Have had sexual partners who are infected or are at risk for infection because they are bisexual or are IV drug abusers or hemophiliacs
- Are living in communities or were born in countries where there is a known or suspected high prevalence of infection among women
- Received a transfusion before blood was being screened for HIV antibody but after HIV infection occurred in the United States (e.g., between 1978 and 1985)

Educating and testing these women before they become pregnant allows them to avoid pregnancy and subsequent intrauterine perinatal infection of their infants (30%-50% of the infants born to HIV-infected women will also be infected).

All pregnant women at risk for HIV infection should be routinely counseled and tested for HIV antibody. Identifying pregnant women with HIV infection as early in pregnancy as possible is important for ensuring appropriate medical care for these women; for planning medical care for their infants; and for providing counseling on family planning, future pregnancies, and the risk of sexual transmission of HIV to others.

All women who seek family planning services and who are at risk for HIV infection should be routinely counseled about AIDS and HIV infection and tested for HIV antibody. Decisions about the need for counseling and testing programs in a community should be based on the best available estimates of the prevalence of HIV infection and the demographic variables of infection.

5. **Persons planning marriage.** All persons considering marriage should be given information about AIDS, HIV infection, and the availability of counseling and testing for HIV antibody. Decisions about instituting routine or mandatory premarital testing for HIV antibody should take into account the prevalence of HIV infection in the area and/or population group as well as other factors and should be based upon the likely cost-effectiveness of such testing

in preventing further spread of infection. Premarital testing in an area with a prevalence of HIV infection as low as 0.1% may be justified if reaching an infected person through testing can prevent subsequent transmission to the spouse or prevent pregnancy in a woman who is infected.

6. **Persons undergoing medical evaluation or treatment.** Testing for HIV antibody is a useful diagnostic tool for evaluating patients with selected clinical signs and symptoms such as generalized lymphadenopathy; unexplained dementia; chronic, unexplained fever or diarrhea; unexplained weight loss; or diseases such as tuberculosis as well as sexually transmitted diseases, generalized herpes, and chronic candidiasis.

Since persons infected with both HIV and the tubercle bacillus are at high risk for severe clinical tuberculosis, all patients with tuberculosis should be routinely counseled and tested for HIV antibody (CDC, 1987c). Guidelines for managing patients with both HIV and tuberculous infection have been published (CDC, 1986b).

The risk of HIV infection from transfusions of blood or blood components from 1978–1985 was greatest for persons receiving large numbers of units of blood collected from areas with high incidences of AIDS. Persons who have this increased risk should be counseled about the potential risk of HIV infection and should be offered antibody testing (CDC, 1987a).

7. **Persons admitted to hospitals.** Hospitals, in conjunction with state and local health departments, should periodically determine the prevalence of HIV infections in the age groups at highest risk for infection. Consideration should be given to routine testing in those age groups deemed to have a high prevalence of HIV infection.

8. **Persons in correctional systems.** Correctional systems should study the best means of implementing programs for counseling inmates about HIV infection and for testing them for such infection at admission and discharge from the system. In particular, they should examine the usefulness of these programs in preventing further transmission of HIV infection and the impact of the testing programs on both the inmates and the correctional system

(Hammett, 1987). Federal prisons have been instructed to test all prisoners when they enter and leave the prison system.

9. **Prostitutes.** Male and female prostitutes should be counseled and tested and made aware of the risks of HIV infection to themselves and others. Particularly prostitutes who are HIV-antibody positive should be instructed to discontinue the practice of prostitution. Local or state jurisdictions should adopt procedures to assure that these instructions are followed.

PARTNER NOTIFICATION/CONTACT TRACING

Sexual partners and those who share needles with HIV-infected persons are at risk for HIV infection and should be routinely counseled and tested for HIV antibody. Persons who are HIV-antibody positive should be instructed in how to notify their partners and to refer them for counseling and testing. If they are unwilling to notify their partners or if it cannot be assured that their partners will seek counseling, physicians or health department personnnel should use confidential procedures to assure that the partners are notified.

CONFIDENTIALITY AND ANTIDISCRIMINATION CONSIDERATIONS

The ability of health departments, hospitals, and other health-care providers and institutions to assure confidentiality of patient information and the public's confidence in that ability are crucial to efforts to increase the number of persons being counseled and tested for HIV infection. Moreover, to assure broad participation in the counseling and testing programs, it is of equal or greater importance that the public perceive that persons found to be positive will not be subject to inappropriate discrimination.

Every reasonable effort should be made to improve confidentiality of test results. The confidentiality of related records can be improved by a careful review of actual recordkeeping practices and by assessing the degree to which these records can be protected under applicable state laws. State laws should be examined and strengthened when found necessary. Because of the wide scope of "need-to-know" situations, because of the possibility of inappropriate disclosures, and because of established authorization procedures for releasing records, it is recognized that there is no perfect solution to confidentiality problems in all situations. Whether disclosures of HIV-testing information are deliberate, inadvertent, or simply unavoidable, public health policy needs to carefully consider ways to reduce the harmful impact of such disclosures.

Public health prevention policy to reduce the transmission of HIV infection can be furthered by an expanded program of counseling and testing for HIV antibody, but the extent to which these programs are successful depends on the level of participation. Persons are more likely to participate in counseling and testing programs if they believe that they will not experience negative consequences in areas such as employment, school admission, housing, and medical services should they test positive. There is no known medical reason to avoid an infected person in these and ordinary social situations since the cumulative evidence is strong that HIV infection is not spread through casual contact. It is essential to the success of counseling and testing programs that persons who are tested for HIV not be subjected to inappropriate discrimination.

REFERENCES

Bayer, R., C. Levine & S. M. Wolf (1986) HIV antibody screening: An ethical framework for evaluating proposed programs. *Journal of the American Medical Association* 256:1768–1774.

Burke, D. S., B. L. Brandt, R. R. Redfield, et al. (1987) Diagnosis of human immunodeficiency virus infection by immunoassay using a molecularly cloned and expressed virus envelope polypeptide. *Annals of Internal Medicine* 106:671–676.

CDC (1986a) Additional recommendations to reduce sexual and drug abuse-related transmission of human T-lymphotropic virus type III/lymphadenopathy-associated virus. *Morbidity and Mortality Report,* 35,152–5.

CDC (1986b) Diagnosis and management of mycobacterial infection and disease in persons with human T-lymphotropic virus type III/lymphadenopathy-associated virus infection. *Morbidity and Mortality Report* 35:448–452.

CDC (1987a) Human immunodeficiency virus infection in transfusion recipients and their family members. *Morbidity and Mortality Report* 36:137–140.

CDC (1987b) *Recommended Additional Guidelines for HIV Antibody Counseling and Testing in the Prevention of HIV Infection and AIDS.* Atlanta: U.S. Department of Health and Human Services, Public Health Service.

CDC (1987c) Tuberculosis provisional data-United States, 1986. *Morbidity and Mortality Report* 36:254–255.

Hammett, T. M. (1987) *AIDS in Correctional Facilities: Issues and Options,* 2d ed. Washington, D.C.: U.S. Department of Justice, National Institute of Justice.

Meyer, K. B. & S. G. Pauker (1987) Screening for HIV: Can we afford the false positive rate? *New England Journal of Medicine* 317:238–241.

APPENDIX D

OSHA Guidelines: Protection Against Occupational Exposure to Hepatitis B Virus (HBV) and Human Immunodeficiency Virus (HIV)

DEPARTMENT OF LABOR
Office of the Secretary

Joint Advisory Notice; Department of Labor/Department of Health and Human Services; HBV/HIV

The Department of Labor hereby gives notice of a joint cover letter and Joint Advisory Notice, entitled "Protection Against Occupational Exposure to Hepatitis B Virus (HBV) and Human Immunodeficiency Virus (HIV)," which will be mailed on or about October 30, 1987 to health-care employers throughout the United States.

The letter and notice are attached hereto and are being mailed to approximately 500,000 employers. Signed at Washington, D.C. this 21st day of October 1987. Michael E. Baroody, Assistant Secretary for Policy, U.S. Department of Labor.

U.S. Department of Labor
Secretary of Labor
Washington, D.C.
October 30, 1987

Dear Health-Care Employer: We are writing to you about a serious health-care problem that faces all Americans but is particularly acute for health-care workers. That problem is potential exposure to hepatitis B virus (HBV), human immune deficiency virus (HIV), which causes

Federal Register 52(210), Friday, October 30, 1987.

acquired immunodeficiency syndrome (AIDS), and other blood-borne diseases.

The Centers for Disease Control (CDC), which is part of the U.S. Department of Health and Human Services (HHS), believes that as many as 18,000 health-care workers per year may be infected by the HBV. Nearly ten percent of those who become infected become long-term carriers of the virus and may have to give up their profession. Several hundred health-care workers will become acutely ill or jaundiced from hepatitis B, and as many as 300 health-care workers may die annually as a result of hepatitis B infections or complication.

Infection with the HIV in the workplace represents a small but real hazard to health-care workers. Fewer than ten cases have been reported to date, but it is not clear that these include all such infections. The CDC expects that with 1.5 million persons now believed to be infected by HIV, the number of AIDS cases in the general population may grow to as many as 270,000 by 1991 from the 40,000 which had been reported by August, 1987. The increases in AIDS cases and in the number of individuals who are infected with the virus will mean an increased potential for exposure to health-care workers.

Fortunately there are reasonable precautions which can be taken by health-care workers to prevent exposure to HBV, HIV, and other blood-borne infectious diseases. Precautions for HBV and HIV have been published by the CDC on several occasions, most recently on June 19, 1987, and on August 21, 1987. The enclosed advisory notice, entitled "Protection Against Occupational Exposure to Hepatitis B Virus (HBV) and Human Immunodeficiency Virus (HIV)," reflects many of the precautions addressed in the CDC guidelines and includes other precautions which should be considered.

It is the legal responsibility of employers to provide appropriate safeguards for health-care workers who may be exposed to these dangerous viruses. For that reason, the Occupational Safety and Health Administration (OSHA) of the U.S. Department of Labor (DOL) is beginning a program of enforcement to insure that health-care employers are meeting those needs. OSHA will respond to employee complaints and conduct other inspections to assure that appropriate measures are being followed. OSHA is currently enforcing its existing regulations and statutory provisions relating to the duty of an employer to provide "safe and healthful working conditions." OSHA is also seeking input about what additional regulatory action may be needed in an Advance Notice of Proposed Rulemaking which will be published in the *Federal Register.*

States with approved plans to operate their own occupational safety and health program enforce standards comparable to the Federal standards and are encouraged to enforce State counterparts to the General Duty Clause. State plan standards, unlike Federal standards, apply to State, county, and municipal workers as well as to private employers.

DOL joins HHS in urging the widest possible adherence to the appropriate precautions as exemplified by the CDC guidelines and the joint advisory notice. All health-care workers who may be exposed to HBV or HIV should receive training and should utilize appropriate precautions.

If you have further questions, please contact your State public health department or OSHA office, or call the Public Health Service National AIDS Hotline, 1-800-342-AIDS. Every effort will be made to respond to your questions in a timely and informative manner. Your unions, and professional and trade associations are also available to answer your questions. We are making every effort to keep all interested parties informed.

The dangers of HBV and HIV are very real, but you can prevent or minimize those dangers for health-care workers through the utilization of the appropriate precautions recommended by the CDC.

Thank you for your time and consideration.

Very truly yours,

William E. Brock, Secretary of Labor

Otis R. Bowen, M. D., Secretary of Health and Human Services

Department of Labor/Department of Health and Human Services—Joint Advisory Notice; Protection Against Occupational Exposure to Hepatitis B Virus (HBV) and Human Immunodeficiency Virus (HIV)

I. BACKGROUND

Hepatitis B (previously called serum hepatitis) is the major infectious occupational health hazard in the health-care industry, and a model for the transmission of bloodborne pathogens. In 1985 the Centers for Disease Control (CDC) estimated that there were over 200,000 cases of hepatitis B virus (HBV) infection in the U.S. each year, leading to 10,000 hospitalizations, 250 deaths due to fulminant hepatitis, 4,000 deaths due to hepatitis-related cirrhosis, and 800 deaths due to hepatitis-related primary liver cancer (CDC, 1985c). More recently the CDC estimated the total number of HBV infections to be 300,000 per year with corresponding increases in numbers of hepatitis-related hospitalizations and deaths (CDC, 1987g). The incidence of reported clinical hepatitis B has been increasing in the United States, from 6.9/100,000 in 1978 to 9.2/100,000 in 1981 and 11.5/100,000 in 1985 (CDC, 1987g). The Hepatitis Branch, CDC, has estimated (unpublished) that 500–600 health-care workers whose job entails exposure to blood are hospitalized annually, with over 200 deaths (12–15 due to fulminant hepatitis, 170–200 from cirrhosis, and 40–50 from liver cancer). Studies indicate that 10% to 40% of health-care or dental workers may show serologic evidence of past or present HBV infection (Palmer, Barash, King & Neil, 1983). Health-care costs for hepatitis B and non-A, non-B hepatitis in health-care workers were estimated to be $10–$12 million annually (Grady & Kane, 1981). A safe, immunogenic, and effective vaccine to prevent hepatitis B has been available since 1982 and is recommended by the CDC for health-care workers exposed to blood and body fluids (CDC, 1982b, 1983b, 1984, 1985c, 1987g). According to unpublished CDC estimates, approximately

30–40% of health-care workers in high-risk settings have been vaccinated to date.

According to the most recent data available from the CDC (1987a), acquired immunodeficiency syndrome (AIDS) was the 13th leading cause of years of potential life lost (82,882 years) in 1984, increasing to 11th place in 1985 (152,595 years). As of August 10, 1987, a cumulative total of 40,051 AIDS cases (of which 558 were pediatric) had been reported to the CDC, with 23,165 (57.8%) of these known to have died (CDC, 1987f). Although occupational HIV infection has been documented, no AIDS case or AIDS-related death is believed to be occupationally related (CDC, 1987e). Spending within the Public Health Service related to AIDS has also accelerated rapidly, from $5.6 million in 1982 to $494 million in 1987, with $791 million requested for 1988. Estimates of average lifetime costs for the care of an AIDS patient have varied considerably, but recent evidence suggests the amount is probably in the range of $50,000 to $75,000.

Infection with either HBV or human immunodeficiency virus (HIV), previously called human T-lymphotropic virus type III/lymphadenopathy-associated virus (HTLVIII/LAV) or AIDS-associated retrovirus (ARV) can lead to a number of life-threatening conditions, including cancer (CDC, 1985c, 1986f, 1987g; Koop, 1986). Therefore, exposure to HBV and HIV should be reduced to the maximum extent feasible by engineering controls, work practices, and protective equipment. (Engineering controls are those methods that prevent or limit the potential for exposure at or near as possible to the point of origin, for example by eliminating a hazard by substitution or by isolating the hazard from the work environment.)

II. MODES OF TRANSMISSION

In the U.S. the major mode of HBV transmission is sexual, both homosexual and heterosexual. Also important is parenteral (entry into the body by a route other than the gastrointestinal tract): transmission by shared needles among intravenous drug abusers and to a lesser extent in needlestick injuries or other exposures of health-care workers to blood. HBV is not transmitted by casual contact, fecal-oral or airborne routes, or by contaminated food or drinking water (CDC, 1985b, 1985c, 1987g). Workers are at risk of HBV infection to the extent they are exposed to blood and other body fluids; employment without that exposure, even in a hospital, carries no greater risk than that for the general population (CDC, 1985c). Thus, the high incidence of HBV infection in some clinical settings is particularly unfortunate because the modes of transmission are well known and readily interrupted by attention to work practices and protective equipment, and because transmission can be prevented by vaccination of those without serologic evidence of previous infection.

Identified risk factors for HIV transmission are essentially identical to those for HBV. Homosexual/bisexual males and male intravenous drug abusers account for 85.4% of all AIDS cases, female intravenous drug abusers for 3.4%, and heterosexual contact for 3.8% (CDC, 1987f). Blood transfusion and treatment of hemophilia-coagulation disorders account for 3.0% of cases, and 1.4% are pediatric cases. In only 3.0% of all AIDS cases has a risk factor not been identified (CDC, 1987f). Like HBV, there is no evidence that HIV is transmitted by casual contact, fecal-oral or airborne routes, or by contaminated food or drinking water (CDC, 1985b; Koop, 1986; Vlahov & Polk, 1987), and barriers to HBV are effective against HIV. Workers are at risk of HIV infection to the extent they are directly exposed to blood and body fluids. Even in groups that presumably have high potential exposure to HIV-contaminated fluids and tissues, e.g., health-care workers specializing in treatment of AIDS patients and the parents, spouse, children, or other persons living with AIDS patients, transmission is recognized as occurring only between sexual partners or as a consequence of mucous-membrane or parenteral (including open-wound) exposure to blood or other body fluids (CDC, 1985b, 1986f, 1987e, 1987h; Gestal, 1987; Vlahov & Polk, 1987).

Despite the similarities in the modes of transmission, the risk of HBV infection in health-care settings far exceeds that for HIV infection (CDC, 1985b; Vlahov & Polk, 1987). For example, it has been estimated (Grady, Lee, Prince, et al., 1978; Seeff, Wright, Zimmerman, et al., 1987; Vlahov & Polk, 1987) that the risk of acquiring HBV infection following puncture with a needle contaminated by an HBV carrier ranges from 6% to 30%—far in excess of the risk of HIV infection under similar circumstances, which the CDC and others estimated to be at less than 1% (CDC, 1985b, 1987e, 1987h).

Health-care workers with documented percutaneous or mucous-membrane exposures to blood or body fluids of HIV-infected patients have been prospectively evaluated to determine the risk of infection after such exposures. As of June 30, 1987, 883 health-care workers have been tested for antibody to HIV in an ongoing surveillance project conducted by CDC (McCray, 1986). Of these, 708 (80%) had percutaneous exposures to blood, and 175 (20%) had a mucous membrane or an open wound contaminated by blood or body fluid. Of 396 health-care workers, each of whom had only a convalescent-phase serum sample obtained and tested 90 days or more post-exposure, one—for whom heterosexual transmission could not be ruled out—was seropositive for HIV antibody. For 425 additional health-care workers, both acute- and convalescent-phase serum samples were obtained and tested; none of 74 health-care workers with non-percutaneous exposures seroconverted, and three (0.9%) of 351 with percutaneous exposures seroconverted. None of these three health-care workers had other documented risk factors for infection.

Two other prospective studies to assess the risk of nosocomial acquisition of HIV infection for health-care workers are ongoing in the United States. As of April 30, 1987, 332 health-care workers with a total of 453 needlestick or mucous-membrane exposures to the blood or other body fluids of HIV-infected patients were tested for HIV antibody at the National Institutes of Health (Henderson, Saah, Zak, et al., 1986). These exposed workers included 103 with needlestick injuries and 229 with mucous-membrane exposures; none had seroconverted. A similar study at the University of California of 129 health-care workers with documented needlestick injuries or mucous-membrane exposures to blood or other body fluids from patients with HIV infection has not identified any seroconversions (Gerberding, Bryant-LeBlanc, Nelson, et al., 1987). Results of a prospective study in the United Kingdom identified no evidence of transmission among 150 health-care workers with parenteral or mucous-membrane exposure to blood or other body fluids, secretions, or excretions from patients with HIV infection (McEvoy, Porter, Mortimer, Simmons & Shanson, 1987).

Following needlestick injuries, two health-care workers contracted HBV but not HIV, and in another instance a health-care worker contracted cryptococcus but not HIV from patients infected with both (Vlahov & Polk, 1987). This risk of infection by HIV and other blood-borne pathogens for which immunization is not available extends to all health-care workers exposed to blood, even those who have been immunized against HBV infection. Effective protection against blood-borne disease requires universal observance of common barrier precautions by all workers with potential exposure to blood, body fluids, and tissues (CDC, 1985b, 1987e).

HIV has been isolated from blood, semen, saliva, tears, urine, vaginal secretions, cerebrospinal fluid, breast milk, and amniotic fluid, but only blood and blood products, semen, vaginal secretions, and possibly breast milk (this needs to be confirmed) have been directly linked to transmission of HIV (CDC, 1985b, 1986a, 1987e). Contact with fluids such as saliva and tears has not been shown to result in infection (CDC, 1985b; Gestal, 1987; Vlahov & Polk, 1987). Although other fluids have not been shown to transmit infection, all body fluids and tissues should be regarded as potentially contaminated by HBV or HIV, and treated as if they were infectious. Both HBV and HIV appear to be incapable of penetrating intact skin, but infection may result from infectious fluids coming into contact with mucous membranes or open wounds (including inapparent lesions) on the skin (CDC, 1987h; Vlahov & Polk, 1987). If a procedure involves the potential for skin contact with blood or mucous membranes, then appropriate barriers to skin contact should be worn, e.g., gloves. Investigations of HBV risks associated with dental and other procedures that might produce particulates in air, e.g., centrifuging and dialysis, indicated that the particulates generated were relatively large droplets (spatter), and not true aerosols of suspended particulates that would represent a risk of inhalation exposure (Bond, 1986; Scarlett, 1986; Petersen, Bond, & Favero, 1979). Thus, if there is the potential for splashes or spatter of blood or fluids, face shields or protective eyewear and surgical masks should be worn. Detailed protective measures for health-care workers have been addressed by the CDC (1982a, 1983a, 1985a, 1985b, 1986a, 1986b, 1986c, 1986d, 1987e; Williams, 1983). These can serve as general guides for the specific groups covered, and for the development of comparable procedures in other working environments.

HIV infection is known to have been transmitted by organ transplants and blood transfusions received from persons who were HIV seronegative at the time of donation (CDC, 1986e, 1987c). Falsely negative serology can be due to improperly performed tests or other laboratory error, or testing in that "window" of time during which a recently infected person is infective but has not yet converted from seronegative to seropositive. Detectable levels of antibodies usually develop within 6 to 12 weeks of infection (CDC, 1987d). A recent report suggesting that this "window" may extend to 14 months is not consistent with other data, and therefore requires confirmation (Ranki, Krohn, Antonen, Allain, Leuther, Franchini & Krohn, 1987). If all body fluids and tissues are treated as infectious, no additional level of worker protection will be gained by identifying seropositive patients or workers. Conversely, if worker protection and work practices were upgraded only following the return of positive HBV or HIV serology, then workers would be inadequately protected during the time required for testing. By producing a false sense of safety with "silent" HBV- or HIV-positive patients, a seronegative test may significantly reduce the level of routine vigilance and result in virus exposure. Furthermore, developing, implementing, and administering a program of routine testing would shift resources and energy away from efforts to assure compliance with infection control procedures. Therefore, routine screening of workers or patients for HIV antibodies will not substantially increase the level of protection for workers above that achieved by adherence to strict infection control procedures.

On the other hand, workers who have had parenteral exposure to fluids or tissues may wish to know whether their own antibody status converts from negative to positive. Such a monitoring program can lead to prophylactic interventions in the case of HBV infection, and CDC has published guidelines on pre- and post-exposure prophylaxis of viral hepatitis (CDC, 1985c, 1987g). Future developments may also allow effective intervention in the case of HIV infection. For the present, post-exposure monitoring for HIV at least can release the affected worker from unnecessary emotional stress if infection did not occur, or allow the affected worker to protect sexual partners in the event infection is detected (CDC, 1987c, 1987e).

III. SUMMARY

The cumulative epidemiologic data indicate that transmission of HBV and HIV requires direct, intimate contact with or parenteral inoculation of blood and blood products, semen, or tissues (CDC, 1985b, 1986a, 1986f, 1987e, 1987h; Vlahov & Polk, 1987). The mere presence of, or casual contact with, an infected person cannot be construed as "exposure" to HBV or HIV. Although the theoretical possibility of rare or low-risk alternative modes of transmission cannot be totally excluded, the only documented occupational risks of HBV and HIV infection are associated with parenteral (including open wound) and mucous membrane exposure to blood and tissues (CDC, 1985b, 1987e, 1987g, 1987h; Vlahov & Polk, 1987). Workers occupationally exposed to blood, body fluids, or tissues can be protected from the recognized risks of HBV and HIV infection by imposing barriers in the form of engineering controls, work practices, and protective equipment that are readily available, commonly used, and minimally intrusive.

IV. RECOMMENDATIONS

General

"Exposure" (or "potential exposure") to HBV and HIV should be defined in terms of actual (or potential) skin, mucous membrane, or parenteral contact with blood, body fluids, and tissues. "Tissues" and "fluids" or "body fluids" should be understood to designate not only those materials from humans, but also potentially infectious fluids and tissues associated with laboratory investigations of HBV or HIV, e.g., organs and excreta from experimental animals, embryonated eggs, tissue or cell cultures and culture media, etc.

As the first step in determining what actions are required to protect worker health, every employer should evaluate all working conditions and the specific tasks that workers are expected to encounter as a consequence of employment. That evaluation should lead to the classification of work-related tasks to one of three categories of potential exposure (figure 1). These categories represent those tasks that require protective equipment to be worn during the task (Category I); tasks that do not require any protective equipment (Category III); and an intermediate grouping of tasks (Category II) that also do not require protective equipment, but that inherently include the predictable job-related requirement to perform Category I tasks unexpectedly or on short notice, so that these persons should have immediate access to some minimal set of protective devices. For example, law enforcement personnel or firefighters may be called upon to perform or assist in first aid or to be potentially exposed in some other way. This exposure classification applies to tasks rather than to individuals, who in the course of their daily activities may move from one exposure category to another as they perform various tasks.

CATEGORY I.   Tasks That Involve Exposure to Blood, Body Fluids, or Tissues.

All procedures or other job-related tasks that involve an inherent potential for mucous membrane or skin contact with blood, body fluids, or tissues, or a potential for spills or splashes of them, are Category I tasks. Use of appropriate protective measures should be required for every employee engaged in Category I tasks.

CATEGORY II. Tasks That Involve No Exposure to Blood, Body Fluids, or Tissues, but Employment May Require Performing Unplanned Category I Tasks.

The normal work routine involves no exposure to blood, body fluids, or tissues, but exposure or potential exposure may be required as a condition of employment. Appropriate protective measures should be readily available to every employee engaged in Category II tasks.

CATEGORY III. Tasks That Involve No Exposure to Blood, Body Fluids, or Tissues, and Category I Tasks Are Not a Condition of Employment.

The normal work routine involves no exposure to blood, body fluids, or tissues (although situations can be imagined or hypothesized under which anyone, anywhere, might encounter potential exposure to body fluids). Persons who perform these duties are not called upon as part of their employment to perform or assist in emergency medical care or first aid or to be potentially exposed in some other way. Tasks that involve handling of implements or utensils, use of public or shared bathroom facilities or telephones, and personal contacts such as handshaking are Category III tasks.

Figure D-1 **EXPOSURE CATEGORIES**

For individual Category I and II tasks, engineering controls, work practices, and protective equipment should be selected after careful consideration, for each specific situation, of the overall risk associated with the task. Some of the factors that should be included in that evaluation of risk are the following:

1. Type of body fluid with which there will or may be contact. Blood is of greater concern than urine.
2. Volume of blood or body fluid likely to be encountered. Hip-replacement surgery can be very bloody while corneal transplantation is almost bloodless.
3. Probability of an exposure taking place. Drawing blood will more likely lead to exposure to blood than will performing a physical examination.
4. Probable route of exposure. Needlestick injuries are of greater concern than contact with soiled linens.
5. Virus concentration in the fluid or tissue. The number of viruses per milliliter of fluid in research laboratory cultures may be orders of magnitude higher than in blood. Similarly, viruses have been less frequently found in such fluids as sweat, tears, urine, and saliva.

Engineering controls, work practices, and protective equipment appropriate to the task being performed are critical to minimize HBV and HIV exposure and to prevent infection. Adequate protection can be assured only if the appropriate controls and equipment are provided and all workers know the applicable work practices and how to properly use the required controls or protective equipment. Therefore, employers should establish a detailed work practices program that includes standard operating procedures (SOPs) for all tasks or work areas having the potential for exposure to fluids or tissues, and a worker education program to assure familiarity with work practices and the ability to use properly the controls and equipment provided.

It is essential for both the patient and the health-care worker to be fully aware of the reasons for the preventive measures used. The health-care worker may incorrectly interpret the work practices and protective equipment as signifying that a task is unsafe. The patient may incorrectly interpret the work practices or protective garb as evidence that the health-care provider knows or believes the patient is infected with HBV or HIV. Therefore, worker education programs should strive to allow workers (and to the extent feasible, clients or patients) to recognize the routine use of appropriate work practices and protective equipment as prudent steps that protect the health of all.

If the employer determines that Category I and II tasks do not exist in the workplace, then no specific personal hygiene or protective measures are required. However, these employers should ensure that workers are aware of the risk factors associated with transmission of HBV and HIV so that they can recognize situations which pose increased potential for exposure to HBV or HIV (Category I tasks) and know how to avoid or minimize personal risk. A comparable level of education is necessary for all citizens. Educational materials such as the Surgeon General's Report can provide much of the needed information (CDC, 1987b; Koop, 1986).

If the employer determines that work-related Category I or II tasks exist, then the following procedures should be implemented.

Administrative

The employer should establish formal procedures to ensure that Category I and II tasks are properly identified, SOPs are developed, and employees who must perform these tasks are adequately trained and protected. If responsibility for implementation of these procedures is delegated to a committee, it should include both management and worker representatives. Administrative activities to enhance worker protection include:

1. Evaluating the workplace to:
   a. Establish categories of risk classification for all routine and reasonably anticipatable job-related tasks.
   b. Identify all workers whose employment requires performance of Category I or II tasks.
   c. Determine for identified Category I and II tasks those body fluids to which workers most probably will be exposed and the potential extent and route of exposure.
2. Developing, or supervising the development of, Standard Operating Procedures (SOPs) for all Category I or II tasks. These SOPs should include mandatory work practices and protective equipment for each Category I or II task.
3. Monitoring the effectiveness of work practices and protective

equipment. This includes:

a. Surveillance of the workplace to ensure that required work practices are observed and that protective clothing and equipment are provided and properly used.

b. Investigation of known or suspected parenteral exposures to body fluids or tissues to establish the conditions surrounding the exposure and to improve training, work practices, or protective equipment to prevent a recurrence.

Training and Education

The employer should establish an initial and periodic training program for all employees who perform Category I and II tasks. No worker should engage in any Category I or II task before receiving training pertaining to the SOPs, work practices, and protective equipment required for that task. The training program should ensure that all workers:

1. Understand the modes of transmission of HBV and HIV.
2. Can recognize and differentiate Category I and II tasks.
3. Know the types of protective clothing and equipment generally appropriate for Category I and II tasks, and understand the basis for selection of clothing and equipment.
4. Are familiar with appropriate actions to take and persons to contact if unplanned-for Category I tasks are encountered.
5. Are familiar with and understand all the requirements for work practices and protective equipment specified in SOPs covering the tasks they perform.
6. Know where protective clothing and equipment is kept, how to use it properly, and how to remove, handle, decontaminate, and dispose of contaminated clothing or equipment.
7. Know and understand the limitations of protective clothing and equipment. For example, ordinary gloves offer no protection against needlestick injuries. Employers and workers should be on guard against a sense of security not warranted by the protective equipment being used.
8. Know the corrective actions to take in the event of spills or personal exposure to fluids or tissues, the appropriate reporting procedures, and the medical monitoring recommended in cases of suspected parenteral exposure.

Engineering Controls

Whenever possible, engineering controls should be used as the primary method to reduce worker exposure to harmful substances. The preferred approach in engineering controls is to use, to the fullest extent feasible, intrinsically safe substances, procedures, or devices. Replacement of a hazardous procedure or device with one that is less risky or harmful is an example of this approach. For example, a laser scalpel reduces the risk of cuts and scrapes by eliminating the necessity to handle the conventional scalpel blade.

Isolation or containment of the hazard is an alternative engineering control technique. Disposable, puncture-resistant containers for used needles, blades, etc., isolate cut and needlestick injury hazards from the worker. Glove boxes, ventilated cabinets, or other enclosures for tissue homogenizers, sonicators, vortex mixers, etc., serve not only to isolate the hazard, but also to contain spills or splashes and prevent spatter and mist from reaching the worker.

After the potential for exposure has been minimized by engineering controls, further reductions can be achieved by work practices and, finally, personal protective equipment.

Work Practices

For all identified Category I and II tasks, the employer should have written, detailed Standard Operating Procedures (SOPs). All employees who perform Category I or II tasks should have ready access to the SOPs pertaining to those tasks.

1. Work practices should be developed on the assumption that all body fluids and tissues are infectious. General procedures to protect health-care workers against HBV or HIV transmission have been published elsewhere (CDC, 1982a; 1983a; 1985a, 1985c, 1986a, 1986c, 1986d, 1987g; Williams, 1983). Each employer with Category I and II tasks in the workplace should incorporate those general recommendations, as appropriate, or equivalent procedures into work practices and SOPs. The importance of handwashing should be emphasized.
2. Work practices should include provision for safe collection of fluids and tissues and for disposal in accordance with applicable local, state, and federal regulations. Provision must be made for

safe removal, handling, and disposal or decontamination of
protective clothing and equipment, soiled linens, etc.

3. Work practices and SOPs should provide guidance on procedures
   to follow in the event of spills or personal exposure to fluids or
   tissues. These procedures should include instructions for personal
   and area decontamination as well as appropriate management or
   supervisory personnel to whom the incident should be reported.
4. Work practices should give specific and detailed procedures to
   be observed with sharp objects, e.g., needles and scalpel blades.
   Puncture-resistant receptacles must be readily accessible for depositing these materials after use. These receptacles must be
   clearly marked and specific work practices provided to protect
   personnel responsible for disposing of them or processing their
   contents for reuse.

Personal Protective Equipment

Based upon the fluid or tissue to which there is potential exposure,
the likelihood of exposure occurring, the potential volume of material,
the probable route of exposure, and overall working conditions and
job requirements, the employer should provide and maintain personal
protective equipment appropriate to the specific requirements of each
task.

For workers performing Category I tasks, a required minimum array
of protective clothing or equipment should be specified by pertinent
SOPs. Category I tasks do not all involve the same type or degree of
risk, and therefore they do not all require the same kind or extent of
protection. Specific combinations of clothing and equipment must be
tailored to specific tasks. Minimum levels of protection for Category I
tasks in most cases would include use of appropriate gloves. If there is
the potential for splashes, protective eyewear or face shields should be
worn. Paramedics responding to an auto accident might protect
against cuts on metal and glass by wearing gloves or gauntlets that are
both puncture-resistant and impervious to blood. If the conditions of
exposure include the potential for clothing becoming soaked with
blood, protective outer garments such as impervious coveralls should
be worn.

For workers performing Category II tasks, there should be ready
access to appropriate protective eyewear, or surgical masks, specified

in pertinent SOPs. Workers performing Category II tasks need not be wearing protective equipment, but they should be prepared to put on appropriate protective garb on short notice.

Medical

In addition to any health care or surveillance required by other rules, regulations, or labor-management agreement, the employer should make available at no cost to the worker:

1. Voluntary HBV immunization for all workers whose employment requires them to perform Category I tasks and who test negative for HBV antibodies. Detailed recommendations for protecting health-care workers from viral hepatitis have been published by the CDC (1985c). These recommendations include procedures for both pre- and post-exposure prophylaxis, and should be the basis for the routine approach by management to the prevention of occupational hepatitis B.
2. Monitoring, at the request of the worker, for HBV and HIV antibodies following known or suspected parenteral exposure to blood, body fluids, or tissues. This monitoring program must include appropriate provisions to protect the confidentiality of test results for all workers who may elect to participate.
3. Medical counseling for all workers found, as a result of the monitoring described above, to be seropositive for HBV or HIV. Counseling guidelines have been published by the Public Health Service (CDC, 1985c, 1987d, 1987g).

Recordkeeping

If any employee is required to perform Category I or II tasks, the employer should maintain records documenting:

1. The administrative procedures used to classify job tasks. Records should describe the factors considered and outline the rationale for classification.
2. Copies of all SOPs for Category I and II tasks, and documentation of the administrative review and approval process through which each SOP passed.

3. Training records, indicating the dates of training sessions, the content of those training sessions along with the names of all persons conducting the training, and the names of all those receiving training.
4. The conditions observed in routine surveillance of the workplace for compliance with work practices and use of protective clothing or equipment. If noncompliance is noted, the conditions should be documented along with corrective actions taken.
5. The conditions associated with each incident of mucous membrane of parenteral exposure to body fluids or tissue, an evaluation of those conditions, and a description of any corrective measures taken to prevent a recurrence or other similar exposure.

REFERENCES

Bond, W. W. (1986) Modes of transmission of infectious diseases. In *Proceedings of the National Conference on Infection Control in Dentistry*, pp. 29–35. Chicago.

Centers for Disease Control (1982a) Acquired immune-deficiency syndrome (AIDS)-Precautions for clinical and laboratory staff. *Morbidity and Mortality Weekly Report* 31:577–580.

Centers for Disease Control (1982b) Hepatitis B virus vaccine safety—Report of an inter-agency group. *Morbidity and Mortality Weekly Report* 31:465–467.

Centers for Disease Control (1983a) Acquired immunodeficiency syndrome (AIDS)—Precautions for health-care workers and allied professionals. *Morbidity and Mortality Weekly Report* 32:450–452.

Centers for Disease Control (1983b) The safety of hepatitis B virus vaccine. *Morbidity and Mortality Weekly Report* 32:134–136.

Centers for Disease Control (1984) Hepatitis B vaccine—Evidence confirming lack of AIDS transmission. *Morbidity and Mortality Weekly Report* 33:685–687.

Centers for Disease Control (1985a) Recommendations for preventing possible transmission of human T-lymphotropic virus type III/lymphadenopathy-associated virus from tears. *Morbidity and Mortality Weekly Report* 34:533–534.

Centers for Disease Control (1985b) Recommendations for preventing transmission of infection with human T-lymphotropic

virus type III/lymphadenopathy-associated virus in the
workplace. *Morbidity and Mortality Weekly Report*
34:681–686, 691–695.

Centers for Disease Control (1985c) Recommendations for protection against viral hepatitis. *Morbidity and Mortality Weekly
Report* 34:313–324, 329–335.

Centers for Disease Control (1986a) Human T-lymphotropic virus,
type III/lymphadenopathy-associated virus—Agent summary
statement. *Morbidity and Mortality Weekly Report*
35:540–542.

Centers for Disease Control (1986b) Recommendations for preventing transmission of infection with human T-lymphotropic
virus type III/lymphadenopathy-associated virus during
invasive procedures. *Morbidity and Mortality Weekly Report*
35:221–223.

Centers for Disease Control (1986c) Recommendations for providing dialysis treatment to patients infected with human T-
lymphotropic virus, type III/lymphadenopathy-associated
virus. *Morbidity and Mortality Weekly Report* 35:376, 383.

Centers for Disease Control (1986d) Recommended infection-
control practices for dentistry. *Morbidity and Mortality
Weekly Report* 35:237–242.

Centers for Disease Control (1986e) Transfusion-associated human
T-lymphotropic virus type III/lymphadenopathy-associated
virus infection from a seronegative donor—Colorado. *Morbidity and Mortality Weekly Report* 35:389–391.

Centers for Disease Control (1986f) Update—Acquired immunodeficiency syndrome—United States. *Morbidity and Mortality
Weekly Report* 35:757–766.

Centers for Disease Control (1987a) Changes in premature mortality—United States, 1984–1985. *Morbidity and Mortality
Weekly Report* 36:55–57.

Centers for Disease Control (1987b) *Facts about AIDS.* U.S. Department of Health and Human Services.

Centers for Disease Control (1987c) Human immunodeficiency
virus infections transmitted from an organ donor screened for
HIV antibody—North Carolina. *Morbidity and Mortality
Weekly Report* 36:306–308.

Centers for Disease Control (1987d) Public Health Service guidelines for counseling and antibody testing to prevent HIV

infection and AIDS. *Morbidity and Mortality Weekly Report* 36:509–515.

Centers for Disease Control (1987e) Recommendations for prevention of HIV transmission in health-care settings. *Morbidity and Mortality Weekly Report* Supplement 36(2S):1S–16S.

Centers for Disease Control (1987f) Update—Acquired immunodeficiency syndrome—United States. *Morbidity and Mortality Weekly Report* Supplement 36:522–526.

Centers for Disease Control (1987g) Update on Hepatitis B prevention. *Morbidity and Mortality Weekly Report* 36:353–360.

Centers for Disease Control (1987h) Update-Human immunodeficiency virus infections in health-care workers exposed to blood of infected patients. *Morbidity and Mortality Weekly Report* 36:285–289.

Gerberding, J. L., C.E. Bryant-LeBlanc, K. Nelson, et al. (1987) Risk of transmitting the human immunodeficiency virus, cytomegalovirus, and hepatitis B virus to health-care workers exposed to patients with AIDS and AIDS-related conditions. *Journal of Infectious Disease* 156:1–8.

Gestal, J. J. (1987) Occupational hazards in hospitals—Risk of infection. *British Journal of Industrial Medicine* 44:435–442.

Grady, G. F. & M. A. Kane (1981) Hepatitis B infections account for multi-million dollar loss. *Hospital Infection Control* 8:60–62.

Grady, G. F., V. A. Lee, A. Prince, et al. (1978) Hepatitis B immune globulin for accidental exposures among medical personnel—Final report of a multicenter controlled trial. *Journal of Infectious Disease* 138:625–638.

Henderson, D. K., A. J. Saah, B. J. Zak, et al. (1986) Risk of nosocomial infection with human T-cell lymphotropic virus type III/lymphadenopathy-associated virus in a large cohort of intensively exposed health-care workers. *Annals of Internal Medicine* 104:644–647.

Koop, C. E. (1986, October). *Surgeon General's Report on Acquired Immune Deficiency Syndrome*. U.S. Department of Health and Human Services.

McCray, E. (1986) The cooperative needlestick surveillance group. Occupational risk of the acquired immunodeficiency syndrome among health-care workers. *New England Journal of Medicine* 314:1127–1132.

McEvoy, M., K. Porter, P. Mortimer, N. Simmons & D. Shanson, (1987) Prospective study of clinical, laboratory, and ancillary staff with accidental exposures to blood or other body fluids from patients infected with HIV. *British Medical Journal* 294:1595–1597.

Palmer, D. L., M. Barash, R. King & F. Neil (1983) Hepatitis among hospital employees. *Western Journal of Medicine* 138:519–523.

Petersen, N. J., W. W. Bond & M. S. Favero (1979) Air sampling for hepatitis B surface antigen in a dental operatory. *Journal of the American Dental Association* 99:465–467.

Ranki, S. L., M. Krohn, J. Antonen, J.P. Allain, M. Leuther, G. Franchini, & K. Krohn(1987) Long latency precedes overt seroconversion in sexually transmitted human-immunodeficiency-virus infection. *Lancet* 2(8559):589–593.

Scarlett, M. (1986) Infection control practices in dentistry. In *Proceedings of the National Conference on Infection Control in Dentistry*, pp. 41–51. Chicago.

Seeff, L. B., E. C. Wright, H. J. Zimmerman, et al. (1987) Type B hepatitis after needlestick exposure—Prevention with hepatitis B immune globulin. *Annals of Internal Medicine* 88:285–293.

Vlahov, D. & B. F. Polk (1987). Transmission of human immunodeficiency virus within the health-care setting. *Occupational Medical State of the Art Reviews* 2:429–450.

Williams, W. W. (1983) Guidelines for infection control in hospital personnel. *Infection Control* 4:326–349.

APPENDIX E

AIDS ORGANIZATIONS AND RESOURCES

AIDS Hotline
800-342-AIDS (U.S. Public
  Health Service)
Operated by the American
  Social Health Association
P.O. Box 13827
Research Triangle Park, NC
27709

AIDS Action Council
729 8th St. SE
Suite 200
Washington, DC 20003
202-293-2886

American Foundation for AIDS
  Research
5900 Wilshire Blvd.
2nd Floor, East Satellite
Los Angeles, CA 90036-5032
(213)857-5900

40 W. 57th Street
Suite 406
New York, NY 10019-4001
(212)333-3118

American Red Cross
AIDS Education Office

1730 E Street NW
Washington, DC 20006
(202) 639-3223

American Social Health
  Association
P. O. Box 13827
Research Triangle Park, NC
27709
(919) 361-4622

Centers for Disease Control
National AIDS Information
  Campaign
1600 Clifton Rd
Atlanta, GA 30029
(404) 639-3298

Gay Men's Health Crisis
Box 274
132 West 24th St.
New York, NY 10011
(212) 807-6655

The Hastings Center Project on
  AIDS, Public Health and
  Civil Liberties
The Hastings Center

255 Elm Road
Briarcliff Manor, NY 10510
(914) 762-8500

Health Education Resource
    Organization (HERO)
101 West Read Street
Suite 819
Baltimore, MD 21201
(301) 685-1180
Hotline: (301) 945-AIDS or
(301) 333-AIDS

Health Resources and Service
    Administration
AIDS Services Branch
5600 Fishers Lane
Rm 913
Rockville, MD 20857
(301) 443-6745

National AIDS Information
    Clearinghouse
P.O. Box 6003
Rockville, MD 20850
*To order AIDS educational
    materials*

National AIDS Network
2033 M Street NW
Suite 800
Washington, DC 20036
(202) 293-2437

National Association of Persons
    with AIDS (PWA)
2025 I Street NW
Suite 415
Washington, DC 20006
(202) 429-2856

National Clearinghouse for
    Alcohol and Drug Information
P.O. Box 2345
Rockville, MD 20852
(301) 468-2600
*Literature on AIDS and
    chemical dependency*

National Council of Churches
AIDS Task Force
475 Riverside Dr.
New York, NY 10015
(212) 870-2511

National Gay Task Force
    AIDS Information Hotline
(800) 221-7044 evenings and
1-5 P.M. Saturdays
(212) 529-1604

National Hemophilia
    Foundation
Soho Building
110 Greene St.
Rm 406
New York, NY 10012
(212) 219-8180

National Institute on Drug
    Abuse (NIDA)
12280 Wilkins Avenue
1st Floor
Rockville, MD 20852
(800) 662-HELP

National Leadership Coalition
    on AIDS
1150 17th St NW
Suite 202
Washington, DC 20036
(202) 429-0930

National Minority AIDS Council
714 G Street SE
Washington, DC 20038
(202) 544-1076

San Francisco AIDS Foundation
333 Valencia Street
P.O. Box 6182
San Francisco, CA 94101-6182
(415) 861-3397

Shanti Project
525 Howard Street
San Francisco, CA 94105
(415) 777-CARE

U.S. Public Health Service
   Hotline
(800) 342-2437 (general)
(800) 447-AIDS (specific
questions)

U.S. Public Service
Public Affairs Office
Hubert Humphrey Building
Room 725-H
200 Independence Ave SW
Washington, DC 20201

EDUCATIONAL RESOURCES

About AIDS in the Workplace
   (pamphlet)
Channing L. Bete Co., Inc.
200 State Road
South Deerfield, MA 01273
(800) 628-7733

AIDS and Religion Resource
   Directory

National Leadership Coalition
   on AIDS
1150 17th St NW
Suite 202
Washington, DC 20036
(202) 429-0930

AIDS and the Law: A Guide for
   the Public (book)
by Dalton, Burris, and the Yale
   AIDS Law Project
Yale University Press
ISBN # 0-300-04078-4

AIDS and the Law Enforcement
   Officer (brochure)
National Institute of Justice
   Reports
U.S. Department of Justice
Box 6000
Rockville, MD 20850

AIDS and the Safety of the
   Nation's Blood Supply
   (pamphlet)
American Red Cross and the
   U.S. Public Health Service.
*Covers information about how
   the blood supply has been
   protected.*

AIDS and Your Job—Are There
   Risks? (brochure)
American Red Cross
AIDS: Corporate America
   Responds
Allstate Insurance Company
Consumer Information
Attn: Public Issues
   Department 10316

P.O. Box 7660
Mount Prospect, IL 60056-9961

AIDS Educator Catalog
San Francisco AIDS Foundation
333 Valencia St.
P.O. Box 6182
San Francisco, CA 94101-6182
*Catalog of videotapes,
pamphlets, posters for AIDS
education*

AIDS Educator: SFAF
P.O. Box 6182
San Francisco, CA 94101-6182
(415) 861-3397

AIDS Fact Book: Everything
You Need to Know to Protect
Yourself and Your Family
AIDS, New Body Health Series,
Volume 1 (1), January 1986.
Available from GCR Publishing
Company, 888 Seventh
Avenue, New York, NY 10106

AIDSFILE (newsletter)
San Francisco General Hospital
Ward 84, 995 Potrero Avenue
San Francisco, CA 94110

AIDS in Children, Adolescents,
and Heterosexual Adults: An
Interdisciplinary Approach to
Prevention (book)
Edited by Raymond Schinazi
and Andre Nahmias.
New York: Elsevier Science
Publishing Co., 1988.

AIDS Information Resources
Directory

American Foundation for AIDS
Research
40 West 57th St.
New York, NY 10019
May 1988 publication

AIDS in the Workplace (video,
manager's guide, appendix)
San Francisco AIDS Foundation
333 Valencia St. 4th Floor
P.O. Box 6182
San Francisco, CA 94101-6182
(415) 861-3397

AIDS in the Workplace (binder)
Bureau of National Affairs
1231 25th St. NW
Washington, DC 20037
(800) 372-1033
Product Code BSP-69

AIDS: Legal Implications for
Health-Care Professionals
(pamphlet)
4455 Woodson Road
St. Louis, MO 63134
*Covers confidentiality, discrim-
ination, employee fears, tort
liability*

AIDS Reference Guide: A
Sourcebook for Planners and
Decisionmakers (book)
Atlantic Information Services
1050 17th St NW
Suite 480
Washington, DC 20036

AIDS: Risk, Prevention, Understanding (brochure)
National Leadership Coalition

on AIDS
1150 17th St NW
Suite 202
Washington, DC 20036
(202) 429-0930

AIDS Service Directory for
  Hispanics (directory)
National Coalition of Hispanic
  Health and Human Service
  Organizations
1030 15th St NW,Suite 1053
Washington, DC 20005

American Association of
  Occupational Health Nurses
  Journal. Special Issue: AIDS
  at the Worksite. July 1988.

And the Band Played On:
  Politics, People and the AIDS
  Epidemic by R. Shilts. New
  York: St. Martin's Press, 1987.

Business Response to AIDS
  (1988 Report)
Fortune Magazine
Rm 1554
1271 Avenue of the Americas
New York, NY 10020

Common Sense about AIDS
  (newsletter)
American Health Consultants
67 Peachtree Park Dr NE
Atlanta, GA 30309-9900
(800) 554-1032
Can be ordered in large
  quantities.

Directory of AIDS Resources: A
  Guide to Sources of

Information
United Way of America
701 North Fairfax Street
Alexandria, VA 22314-2045
(703) 836-7100

Don't Listen to Rumors About
  AIDS. Get the Facts. (poster)
American Red Cross
Stock no. 329510.

Face to Face on AIDS (video-
  based training program)
Corporate Health Policies
  Group
4545 42nd St NW
Suite 109
Washington, DC 20016
(800) 232-HELP
(202) 686-2012

Facilitating AIDS Education in
  the Work Environment
  (manual)
Pacific Financial Companies
Product Information Office—4
P.O. Box 9000
Newport Beach, CA
92658-9952

Facts About AIDS and Drug
  Abuse (pamphlet)
American Red Cross and U. S.
  Public Health Service.
For people who use drugs or
  for partners of drug users.
Call local Red Cross chapter or
  write to:
American Red Cross
National Headquarters
AIDS Public Education Program

1730 D Street, NW
Washington, DC 20006
(202) 639-3223

Focus: A Review of AIDS
  Research (Newsletter)
University of California San
  Francisco AIDS Health
  Project
Box 0884
San Francisco, CA 94143-0884

HIV/AIDS Infection in the
  Workplace (Resource Guide)
American Association of
  Occupational Health Nurses
50 Lenox Pointe
Atlanta, GA 30324

If Your Test for Antibody to the
  AIDS Virus is Positive
  (Pamphlet).
American Red Cross and U. S.
  Public Health Service.
*Information for persons who
  have tested positive for AIDS
  antibodies.*

Local AIDS-Related Services:
  The National Directory
Published in February, 1988
The U.S. Conference of Mayors
1620 I Street, NW
Washington, DC 20006
(202) 293-7330

Managing AIDS in the
  Workplace: An Executive
  Briefing and Training Manual.
Workplace Health

Communications Corporation
4 Madison Place
Albany, NY 12203
(800) 334-4911
In New York, call collect (518)
434-2381
*Contains guidelines for devel-
  oping policies and
  educational programs.*

Morbidity and Mortality Report
Prepared by the Centers for
  Disease Control
U. S. Public Health Service
Atlanta, GA 30333

Paid subscriptions available
from either the Superintendent
of Documents, U.S. Government Printing Office, Washington DC 20402, (202) 783-3238,
or from the Massachusetts Medical Society, C.S.P.O. Box 9120,
Waltham, MA 02254-9120.
Rates: Third class mail $26/
year for 52 issues and supplement; first class mail $46/year.

National and International
  Directory of AIDS Related
  Services
Shanti Project
525 Howard Street
San Francisco, CA 94105
(415) 777-CARE

National AIDS Network
  Directory of AIDS Education
  and Service Organizations
National AIDS Network

1110 Vermont Ave NW,
Suite 550
Washington, DC 20005
(202) 293-2437

Safe Sex for Men and Women
  Concerned about AIDS
  (Pamphlet)
Health Education Resource
  Organization HERO
(800) 638-6252.
In Washington DC, call
  251-1164

Sexual Health Report
  (newsletter)
National Coalition of Gay
  Sexually Transmitted Disease
  Services
c/o Mark Behar
P.O. Box 239
Milwaukee, WI 53201
(414) 277-7671

Shanti Training Project
  (videotape program)
Shanti Project
525 Howard Street
San Francisco, CA 94105
(415) 777-CARE
*40 hour videotape program to
  train laypersons to provide
  support for persons with AIDS.*

The National AIDS Awareness
  Test (video)
Metropolitan Life Insurance Co.
Department 300
One Madison Avenue
New York, NY 10010

The Workplace and AIDS
  (directory)
Personnel Journal
245 Fischer Ave B-2
Costa Mesa, CA 92626

Teens and AIDS: Playing it Safe
  (brochure)
Education Relations and
  Resources.
American Council of Life
  Insurance.
Health Insurance Corporation
  of America.

Understanding AIDS: A
  Message from the Surgeon
  General (brochure)
U.S. Department of Health and
  Human Services
Public Health Service
Centers for Disease Control
P.O. Box 6003
Rockville, MD 20850

Understanding and Preventing
  AIDS (pamphlet)
Krames Communications
312 90th Street
Daly City, CA 94015-1898
*Colorful and appropriate for
  workplace distribution.
  Available in quantity.*

Working Beyond Fear
  (videotape)
American Red Cross
33 minutes. *Includes 3
  workplace scenarios.*

APPENDIX F

CDC Recommendations for Prevention of HIV Transmission in Health-Care Settings

INTRODUCTION

Human immunodeficiency virus (HIV), the virus that causes acquired immunodeficiency syndrome (AIDS), is transmitted through sexual contact and exposure to infected blood or blood components and perinatally from mother to neonate. HIV has been isolated from blood, semen, vaginal secretions, saliva, tears, breast milk, cerebrospinal fluid, amniotic fluid, and urine and is likely to be isolated from other body fluids, secretions, and excretions. However, epidemiologic evidence has implicated only blood, semen, vaginal secretions, and possibly breast milk in transmission.

The increasing prevalence of HIV increases the risk that health-care workers will be exposed to blood from patients infected with HIV, especially when blood and body fluid precautions are not followed for all patients. Thus, this document emphasizes the need for health-care workers to consider all patients as potentially infected with HIV and/or other blood-borne pathogens and to adhere rigorously to infection-control precautions for minimizing the risk of exposure to blood and body fluids of all patients.

The recommendations contained in this document consolidate and update CDC recommendations published earlier for preventing HIV transmission in health-care settings: precautions for clinical and laboratory staffs (CDC, 1982) and precautions for health-care workers and allied professionals (CDC, 1983a); recommendations for preventing HIV transmission in the workplace (CDC, 1985c) and during invasive

Morbidity and Mortality Weekly Report 1987, 36 (Suppl. no. 2S):3S–18S.

procedures (CDC, 1986c); recommendations for preventing possible transmission of HIV from tears (CDC, 1985b); and recommendations for providing dialysis treatment for HIV-infected patients (CDC, 1986d). These recommendations also update portions of the "Guideline for Isolation Precautions in Hospitals" (Garner & Simmons, 1983) and reemphasize some of the recommendations contained in "Infection Control Practices for Dentistry" (CDC, 1986e). The recommendations contained in this document have been developed for use in health-care settings and emphasize the need to treat blood and other body fluids from all patients as potentially infective. These same prudent precautions also should be taken in other settings in which persons may be exposed to blood or other body fluids.

DEFINITION OF HEALTH-CARE WORKERS

Health-care workers are defined as persons, including students and trainees, whose activities involve contact with patients or with blood or other body fluids from patients in a health-care setting.

HEALTH-CARE WORKERS WITH AIDS

As of July 10, 1987, a total of 1,875 (5.8% of 32,395) adults with AIDS, who had been reported to the CDC national surveillance system and for whom occupational information was available, reported being employed in a health-care or clinical laboratory setting. In comparison, 6.8 million persons—representing 5.6% of the U.S. labor force—were employed in health services. Of the health-care workers with AIDS, 95% have been reported to exhibit high-risk behavior; for the remaining 5%, the means of HIV acquisition was undetermined. Health-care workers with AIDS were significantly more likely than other workers to have an undetermined risk (5% versus 3%, respectively). For both health-care workers and non-health-care workers with AIDS, the proportion with an undetermined risk has not increased since 1982.

AIDS patients initially reported as not belonging to recognized risk groups are investigated by state and local health departments to determine whether possible risk factors exist. Of all health-care workers with AIDS reported to CDC who were initially characterized as not having an identified risk and for whom follow-up information was available, 66% have been reclassified because risk factors were identified or because the patient was found not to meet the surveillance case definition for AIDS. Of the 87 health-care workers currently categorized as having no identifiable risk, information is incomplete on 16 (18%) because of death or refusal to be interviewed; 38 (44%) are still being investigated. The remaining 33 (38%) health-care workers were interviewed or had other follow-up information available. The occupations of these 33 were as follows: five physicians (15%), three of whom were surgeons; one dentist (3%), three nurses (9%), nine nursing assistants (27%), seven housekeeping or maintenance workers (21%); three clinical laboratory technicians (9%); one therapist (3%); and four others who did not have contact with patients (12%). Although 15 of these 33 health-care workers reported parenteral and/or other non-needlestick exposure to blood or body fluids from patients in the 10 years preceding their diagnosis of AIDS, none of these exposures involved a patient with AIDS or known HIV infection.

RISK TO HEALTH-CARE WORKERS OF ACQUIRING HIV IN HEALTH-CARE SETTINGS

Health-care workers with documented percutaneous or mucous-membrane exposures to blood or body fluids of HIV-infected patients have been prospectively evaluated to determine the risk of infection after such exposures. As of June 30, 1987, 883 health-care workers have been tested for antibody to HIV in an ongoing surveillance project conducted by CDC (McCray, 1986). Of these 708 (80%) had percutaneous exposures to blood, and 175 (20%) had a mucous membrane or an open wound contaminated by blood or body fluid. Of 396 health-care workers, each of whom had only a convalescent-phase serum sample obtained and tested greater than 90 days post-exposure, one—for whom heterosexual transmission could not be ruled out—was seropositive for HIV antibody. For 425 additional health-care workers, both acute- and convalescent-phase serum samples were obtained and tested; none of 74 health-care workers with nonpercutaneous exposures seroconverted, and three (0.9%) of 351 with percutaneous exposures seroconverted. None of these three health-care workers had other documented risk factors for infection.

Two other prospective studies to assess the risk of nosocomial acquisition of HIV infection for health-care workers are ongoing in the United States. As of April 30, 1987, 332 health-care workers with a total of 453 needlestick or mucous-membrane exposures to the blood or other body fluids of HIV-infected patients were tested for HIV antibody at the National Institutes of Health (Henderson, Saah, Zak, et al., 1986). These exposed workers included 103 with needlestick injuries and 229 with mucous-membrane exposures; none had seroconverted. A similar study at the University of California of 129 health-care workers with documented needlestick injuries or mucousmembrane exposures to blood or other body fluids from patients with HIV infection has not identified any seroconversions (Gerberding, Bryant-LeBlanc, Nelson, et al., 1987). Results of a prospective study in the United Kingdom identified no evidence of transmission among 150 health-care workers with parenteral or mucous-membrane exposures to blood or other body fluids, secretions, or excretions from patients with HIV infection (McEvoy, Porter, Mortimer, Simmons & Shanson, 1987).

In addition to health-care workers enrolled in prospective studies, eight persons who provided care to infected patients and denied other risk factors have been reported to have acquired HIV infection. Three of these health-care workers had needlestick exposures to blood from infected patients (Anonymous, 1984; Neisson-Vernant, Arfi, Mathez, Leibowitch & Monplaisir, 1986; Oksenhendler, Harzic, Le Roux, Rabian, & Clauvel, 1986). Two were persons who provided nursing care to infected persons; although neither sustained a needlestick, both had extensive contact with blood or other body fluids, and neither observed recommended barrier precautions (CDC, 1986a; Grint & McEvoy, 1985). The other three were health-care workers with non-needlestick exposures to blood from infected patients (CDC, 1987b). Although the exact route of transmission for these last three infections is not known, all three persons had direct contact of their skin with blood from infected patients, all had skin lesions that may have been contaminated by blood, and one also had a mucous-membrane exposure.

A total of 1,231 dentists and hygienists, many of whom practiced in areas with many AIDS cases, participated in a study to determine the prevalence of antibody to HIV; one dentist (0.1%) had HIV antibody. Although no exposure to a known HIV-infected person could be documented, epidemiologic investigation did not identify any other risk factor for infection. The infected dentist, who also had a history of sustaining needlestick injuries and trauma to his hands, did not routinely wear gloves when providing dental care (Kline, Phelan, Friedland, et al., 1985).

PRECAUTIONS TO PREVENT TRANSMISSION OF HIV

Universal Precautions

Since medical history and examination cannot reliably identify all patients infected with HIV or other blood-borne pathogens, blood and body-fluid precautions should be consistently used for all patients. This approach, previously recommended by CDC (1985, 1986), and referred to as "universal blood and body-fluid precautions" or "universal precautions," should be used in the care of all patients, especially including those in emergency-care settings in which the risk of blood exposure is increased and the infection status of the patient is usually unknown (Baker, Kelen, Sivertson, & Quinn, 1987).

1. All health-care workers should routinely use appropriate barrier precautions to prevent skin and mucous-membrane exposure when contact with blood or other body fluids of any patient is anticipated. Gloves should be worn for touching blood and body fluids, mucous membranes, or non-intact skin of all patients, for handling items or surfaces soiled with blood or body fluids, and for performing venipuncture and other vascular access procedures. Gloves should be changed after contact with each patient. Masks and protective eyewear or face shields should be worn during procedures that are likely to generate droplets of blood or other body fluids to prevent exposure of mucous membranes of the mouth, nose, and eyes. Gowns or aprons should be worn during procedures that are likely to generate splashes of blood or other body fluids.
2. Hands and other skin surfaces should be washed immediately and thoroughly if contaminated with blood or other body fluids. Hands should be washed immediately after gloves are removed.
3. All health-care workers should take precautions to prevent injuries caused by needles, scalpels, and other sharp instruments or devices during procedures; when cleaning used instruments;

during disposal of used needles; and when handling sharp instruments after procedures. To prevent needlestick injuries, needles should not be recapped, purposely bent or broken by hand, removed from disposable syringes, or otherwise manipulated by hand. After they are used, disposable syringes and needles, scalpel blades, and other sharp items should be placed in puncture-resistant containers for disposal; the puncture-resistant containers should be located as close as practical to the use area. Large-bore reusable needles should be placed in a puncture-resistant container for transport to the reprocessing area.

4. Although saliva has not been implicated in HIV transmission, to minimize the need for emergency mouth-to-mouth resuscitation, mouthpieces, resuscitation bags, or other ventilation devices should be available for use in areas in which the need for resuscitation is predictable.

5. Health-care workers who have exudative lesions or weeping dermatitis should refrain from all direct patient care and from handling patient-care equipment until the condition resolves.

6. Pregnant health-care workers are not known to be at greater risk of contracting HIV infection than health-care workers who are not pregnant; however, if a health-care worker develops HIV infection during pregnancy, the infant is at risk of infection resulting from perinatal transmission. Because of this risk, pregnant health-care workers should be especially familiar with and strictly adhere to precautions to minimize the risk of HIV transmission.

Implementation of universal blood and body-fluid precautions for *all* patients eliminated the need for use of the isolation category of "Blood and Body Fluid Precautions" previously recommended by CDC for patients known or suspected to be infected with blood-borne pathogens (Garner & Simmons, 1983). Isolation precautions (e.g., enteric, "AFB") should be used as necessary if associated conditions, such as infectious diarrhea or tuberculosis, are diagnosed or suspected.

PRECAUTIONS FOR INVASIVE PROCEDURES

In this document, an invasive procedure is defined as surgical entry into tissues, cavities, or organs or repair of major traumatic injuries

(1) in an operating or delivery room, emergency department, or out-patient setting, including both physicians' and dentists' offices; (2) cardiac catheterization and angiographic procedures; (3) a vaginal or cesarean delivery or other invasive obstetric procedure during which bleeding may occur; or (4) the manipulation, cutting, or removal of any oral or perioral tissues, including tooth structure, during which bleeding occurs or the potential for bleeding exists. The universal blood and body-fluid precautions listed above, combined with the precautions listed below, should be the minimum precautions for *all* such invasive procedures.

1. All health-care workers who participate in invasive procedures must routinely use appropriate barrier precautions to prevent skin and mucous-membrane contact with blood and other body fluids of all patients. Gloves and surgical masks must be worn for all invasive procedures. Protective eyewear or face shields should be worn for procedures that commonly result in the generation of droplets, splashing of blood or other body fluids, or the generation of bone chips. Gowns or aprons made of materials that provide an effective barrier should be worn during invasive pro-cedures that are likely to result in the splashing of blood or other body fluids. All health-care workers who perform or assist in vaginal or cesarean deliveries should wear gloves and gowns when handling the placenta or the infant until blood and amniotic fluid have been removed from the infant's skin and should wear gloves during post-delivery care of the umbilical cord.
2. If a glove is torn or a needlestick or other injury occurs, the glove should be removed and a new glove used as promptly as patient safety permits; the needle or instrument involved in the incident should be removed from the sterile field.

PRECAUTIONS FOR DENTISTRY

Blood, saliva, and gingival fluid from all dental patients should be considered infective. Special emphasis should be placed on the following precautions for preventing transmission of blood-borne pathogens in dental practice in both institutional and non-institutional settings.

1. In addition to wearing gloves for contact with oral mucous membranes of all patients, all dental workers should wear surgical masks and protective eyewear or chin-length plastic face shields during dental procedures in which splashing or spattering of blood, saliva, or gingival fluids is likely. Rubber dams, high-speed evacuation, and proper patient positioning, when appropriate, should be utilized to minimize generation of droplets and spatter.
2. Handpieces should be sterilized after use with each patient, since blood, saliva, or gingival fluid of patients may be aspirated into the handpiece or waterline. Handpieces that cannot be sterilized should at least be flushed, the outside surface cleaned and wiped with suitable chemical germicide, and then rinsed. Handpieces should be flushed at the beginning of the day and after use with each patient. Manufacturers' recommendations should be followed for use and maintenance of waterlines and check valves and for flushing of handpieces. The same precautions should be used for ultrasonic scalers and air/water syringes.
3. Blood and saliva should be thoroughly and carefully cleaned from material that has been used in the mouth (e.g., impression materials, bite registration), especially before polishing and grinding intra-oral devices. Contaminated materials, impressions, and intra-oral devices should also be cleaned and disinfected before being handled in the dental laboratory and before they are placed in the patient's mouth. Because of the increasing variety of dental materials used intra-orally, dental workers should consult with manufacturers as to the stability of specific materials when using disinfection procedures.
4. Dental equipment and surfaces that are difficult to disinfect (e.g., light handles or X-ray-unit heads) and that may become contaminated should be wrapped with impervious-backed paper, aluminum foil, or clear plastic wrap. The coverings should be removed and discarded, and clean coverings should be put in place after use with each patient.

PRECAUTIONS FOR AUTOPSIES OR MORTICIANS' SERVICES

In addition to the universal blood and body-fluid precautions listed above, the following precautions should be used by persons performing postmortem procedures:

1. All persons performing or assisting in postmortem procedures should wear gloves, masks, protective eyewear, gowns, and waterproof aprons.
2. Instruments and surfaces contaminated during postmortem procedures should be decontaminated with an appropriate chemical germicide.

PRECAUTIONS FOR DIALYSIS

Patients with end-stage renal disease who are undergoing maintenance dialysis and who have HIV infection can be dialyzed in hospital-based or free-standing dialysis units using conventional infection-control precautions (Favero, 1985). Universal blood and body-fluid precautions should be used when dialyzing all patients.

Strategies for disinfecting the dialysis fluid pathways of the hemodialysis machine are targeted to control bacterial contamination and generally consist of using 500–750 parts per million (ppm) of sodium hypochlorite (household bleach) for 30–40 minutes or 1.5%–2.0% formaldehyde overnight. In addition, several chemical germicides formulated to disinfect dialysis machines are commercially available. None of these protocols or procedures need to be changed for dialyzing patients infected with HIV.

Patients infected with HIV can be dialyzed by either hemodialysis or peritoneal dialysis and do not need to be isolated from other patients. The type of dialysis treatment (i.e., hemodialysis or peritoneal dialysis) should be based on the needs of the patient. The dialyzer may be discarded after each use. Alternatively, centers that reuse dialyzers—i.e., a specific single-use dialyzer is issued to a specific patient, removed, cleaned, disinfected, and reused several times on the same patient only—may include HIV-infected patients in the dialyzer-reuse program. An individual dialyzer must never be used on more than one patient.

PRECAUTIONS FOR LABORATORIES

Blood and other body fluids from all patients should be considered infective. To supplement the universal blood and body-fluid precautions listed above, the following precautions are recommended for health-care workers in clinical laboratories:

1. All specimens of blood and body fluids should be put in a well-constructed container with a secure lid to prevent leaking during transport. Care should be taken when collecting each specimen to avoid contaminating the outside of the container and of the laboratory form accompanying the specimen.
2. All persons processing blood and body-fluid specimens (e.g., removing tops from vacuum tubes) should wear gloves. Masks and protective eyewear should be worn if mucous-membrane contact with blood or body fluids is anticipated. Gloves should be changed and hands washed after completion of specimen processing.
3. For routine procedures, such as histologic and pathologic studies or microbiologic culturing, a biological safety cabinet is not necessary. However, biological safety cabinets (Class I or II) should be used whenever procedures are conducted that have a high potential for generating droplets. These include activities such as blending, sonicating, and vigorous mixing.
4. Mechanical pipetting devices should be used for manipulating all liquids in the laboratory. Mouth pipetting must not be done.
5. Use of needles and syringes should be limited to situations in which there is no alternative, and the recommendations for preventing injuries with needles outlined under universal precautions should be followed.
6. Laboratory work surfaces should be decontaminated with an appropriate chemical germicide after a spill of blood or other body fluids and when work activities are completed.
7. Contaminated materials used in laboratory tests should be decontaminated before reprocessing or be placed in bags and disposed of in accordance with institutional policies for disposal of infective waste.
8. Scientific equipment that has been contaminated with blood or other body fluids should be decontaminated and cleaned before being repaired in the laboratory or transported to the manufacturer.
9. All persons should wash their hands after completing laboratory activities and should remove protective clothing before leaving the laboratory.

Implementation of universal blood and body-fluid precautions for all patients eliminates the need for warning labels on specimens since blood and other body fluids from all patients should be considered infective.

ENVIRONMENTAL CONSIDERATIONS FOR
HIV TRANSMISSION

No environmentally mediated mode of HIV transmission has been documented. Nevertheless, the precautions described below should be taken routinely in the care of all patients.

Sterilization and Disinfection

Standard sterilization and disinfection procedures for patient-care equipment currently recommended for use (Favero, 1985; Garner & Favero, 1985) in a variety of health-care settings—including hospitals, medical and dental clinics and offices, hemodialysis centers, emergency-care facilities, and long-term nursing-care facilities—are adequate to sterilize or disinfect instruments, devices, or other items contaminated with blood or other body fluids from persons infected with blood-borne pathogens including HIV (CDC, 1986b; Favero, 1985).

Instruments or devices that enter sterile tissue or the vascular system of any patient or through which blood flows should be sterilized before reuse. Devices or items that contact intact mucous membranes should be sterilized or receive high-level disinfection, a procedure that kills vegetative organisms and viruses but not necessarily large numbers of bacterial spores. Chemical germicides that are registered with the U.S. Environmental Protection Agency (EPA) as "sterilants" may be used either for sterilization or for high-level disinfection depending on contact time.

Contact lenses used in trial fittings should be disinfected after each fitting by using a hydrogen peroxide contact lens disinfecting system or, if compatible, with heat (78 C–80 C [172.4 F–176.0F]) for 10 minutes.

Medical devices or instruments that require sterilization or disinfection should be thoroughly cleaned before being exposed to the germicide, and the manufacturer's instructions for the use of the germicide should be followed. Further, it is important that the manufacturer's specifications for compatibility of the medical device with chemical germicides be closely followed. Information on specific label claims of commercial germicides can be obtained by writing to the Disinfectants Branch, Office of Pesticides, Environmental Protection Agency, 401 M Street, SW, Washington, DC 20406.

Studies have shown that HIV is inactivated rapidly after being exposed to commonly used chemical germicides at concentrations that are much lower than used in practice (Martin, McDougal & Loskoski, 1985; McDougal, Martin, Cort, et al., 1985; Spire, Barre-Sinoussi, Dormont, Montagnier & Chermann, 1985; Spire, Montagnier, Barre-Sinoussi, & Chermann, 1984). Embalming fluids are similar to the types of chemical germicides that have been tested and found to completely inactivate HIV. In addition to commercially available chemical germicides, a solution of sodium hypochlorite (household bleach) prepared daily is an inexpensive and effective germicide. Concentrations ranging from approximately 500 ppm (1:10 dilution of household bleach) are effective depending on the amount of organic material (e.g., blood, mucus) present on the surface to be cleaned and disinfected. Commercially available chemical germicides may be more compatible with certain medical devices that might be corroded by repeated exposure to sodium hypochlorite, especially to the 1:10 dilution.

SURVIVAL OF HIV IN THE ENVIRONMENT

The most extensive study on the survival of HIV after drying involved greatly concentrated HIV samples, i.e., 10 million tissue-culture infectious doses per milliliter (Resnick, Veren, Salahuddin, Tondreau, & Markham, 1986). This concentration is at least 100,000 times greater than that typically found in the blood or serum of patients with HIV infection. HIV was detectable by tissue-culture techniques 1-3 days after drying, but the rate of inactivation was rapid. Studies performed at CDC have also shown that drying HIV causes a rapid (within several hours) 1-2 log (90%-99%) reduction in HIV concentration. In tissue-culture fluid, cell-free HIV could be detected up to 15 days at room temperature, up to 11 days at 37 C (98.6F), and up to 1 day if the HIV was cell-associated.

When considered in the context of environmental conditions in health-care facilities, these results do not require any changes in currently recommended sterilization, disinfection, or housekeeping strategies. When medical devices are contaminated with blood or other body fluids, existing recommendations include the cleaning of these instruments, followed by disinfection or sterilization, depending on the type of medical device. These protocols assume "worst-case" conditions of extreme virologic and microbiologic contamination, and whether viruses have been inactivated after drying plays no role in formulating these strategies. Consequently, no changes in published procedures for cleaning, disinfecting, or sterilizing need to be made.

HOUSEKEEPING

Environmental surfaces such as walls, floors, and other surfaces are not associated with transmission of infections to patients or health-care workers. Therefore, extraordinary attempts to disinfect or sterilize these environmental surfaces are not necessary. However, cleaning and removal of soil should be done routinely.

Cleaning schedules and methods vary according to the area of the hospital or institution, type of surface to be cleaned, and the amount and type of soil present. Horizontal surfaces (e.g., bedside tables and hard-surfaced flooring) in patient-care areas are usually cleaned on a regular basis, when soiling or spills occur, and when a patient is discharged. Cleaning of walls, blinds, and curtains is recommended only if they are visibly soiled. Disinfectant fogging is an unsatisfactory method of decontaminating air and surfaces and is not recommended.

Disinfectant-detergent formulations registered by EPA can be used for cleaning environmental surfaces, but the actual physical removal of microorganisms by scrubbing is probably at least as important as any antimicrobial effect of the cleaning agent used. Therefore, cost, safety, and acceptability by housekeepers can be the main criteria for selecting any such registered agent. The manufacturers' instructions for appropriate use should be followed.

CLEANING AND DECONTAMINATING SPILLS OF BLOOD OR OTHER BODY FLUIDS

Chemical germicides that are approved for use as "hospital disinfectants" and are tuberculocidal when used at recommended dilutions can be used to decontaminate spills of blood and other body fluids. Strategies for decontaminating spills of blood and other body fluids in a patient-care setting are different than for spills of cultures or other materials in clinical, public health, or research laboratories. In patient-care areas, visible material should first be removed and then the area should be decontaminated. With large spills of cultured or concentrated infectious agents in the laboratory, the contaminated area should be flooded with a liquid germicide before cleaning, then decontaminated with fresh germicidal chemical. In both settings, gloves should be worn during the cleaning and decontaminating procedures.

LAUNDRY

Although soiled linen has been identified as a source of large numbers of certain pathogenic microorganisms, the risk of actual disease transmission is negligible. Rather than rigid procedures and specifications, hygienic and common-sense storage and processing of clean and soiled linen are recommended (Garner & Favero, 1985). Soiled linen should be handled as little as possible and with minimum agitation to prevent gross microbial contamination of the air and of persons handling the linen. All soiled linen should be bagged at the location where it was used; it should not be sorted or rinsed in patient-care areas. Linen soiled with blood or body fluids should be placed and transported in bags that prevent leakage. If hot water is used, linen should be washed with detergent in water at least 71 C (160 F) for 25 minutes. If low-temperature (less than 70 C [148 F]) laundry cycles are used, chemicals suitable for low-temperature washing at proper use concentration should be used.

INFECTIVE WASTE

There is no epidemiologic evidence to suggest that most hospital waste is any more infective than residential waste. Moreover, there is no epidemiologic evidence that hospital waste has caused disease in the community as a result of improper disposal. Therefore, identifying wastes for which special precautions are indicated is largely a matter of judgment about the relative risk of disease transmission. The most practical approach to the management of infective waste is to identify those wastes with the potential for causing infection during handling and disposal and for which some special precautions appear prudent. Hospital wastes for which special precautions appear prudent include microbiology laboratory waste, pathology waste, and blood specimens or blood products. While any item that has had contact with blood, exudates, or secretions may be potentially infective, it is not usually considered practical or necessary to treat all such waste as infective (Environmental Protection Agency, 1986b; Garner & Favero, 1985). Infective waste, in general, should either be incinerated or should be autoclaved before disposal in a sanitary landfill. Bulk blood, suctioned fluids, excretions, and secretions may be carefully poured down a drain connected to a sanitary sewer. Sanitary sewers may also be used to dispose of other infectious wastes capable of being ground and flushed into the sewer.

IMPLEMENTATION OF RECOMMENDED PRECAUTIONS

Employers of health-care workers should ensure that policies exist for:

1. Initial orientation and continuing education and training of all health-care workers—including students and trainees—on the epidemiology, modes of transmission, and prevention of HIV and other blood-borne infections and the need for routine use of universal blood and body-fluid precautions for all patients.
2. Provision of equipment and supplies necessary to minimize the risk of infection with HIV and other blood-borne pathogens.
3. Monitoring adherence to recommended protective measures. When monitoring reveals a failure to follow recommended precautions, counseling, education, and/or re-training should be provided, and, if necessary, appropriate disciplinary action should be considered.

Professional associations and labor organizations, through continuing education efforts, should emphasize the need for health-care workers to follow recommended precautions.

SEROLOGIC TESTING FOR HIV INFECTION

Background

A person is identified as infected with HIV when a sequence of tests, starting with repeated enzyme immunoassays (EIA) and including a Western blot or similar, more specific assay, are repeatedly reactive. Persons infected with HIV usually develop antibody against the virus within 6–12 weeks after infection.

The sensitivity of the currently licensed EIA tests is at least 99% when they are performed under optimal laboratory conditions on serum specimens from persons infected for greater than or equal to 12 weeks. Optimal laboratory conditions include the use of reliable reagents, provision of continuing education of personnel, quality control of procedures, and participation in performance-evaluation programs. Given this performance, the probability of a false-negative test is remote except during the first several weeks after infection, before detectable antibody is present. The proportion of infected persons with a false-negative test attributed to absence of antibody in the early stages of infection is dependent on both the incidence and prevalence of HIV infection in a population.

The specificity of the currently licensed EIA tests is approximately 99% when repeatedly reactive tests are considered. Repeat testing of initially reactive specimens by EIA is required to reduce the likelihood of laboratory error. To increase further the specificity of serologic tests, laboratories must use a supplemental test, most often the Western blot, to validate repeatedly reactive EIA results. Under optimal laboratory conditions, the sensitivity of the Western blot test is comparable to or greater than that of a repeatedly reactive EIA, and the Western blot is highly specific when strict criteria are used to interpret the test results. The testing sequence of a repeatedly reactive EIA and a positive Western blot test is highly predictive of HIV infection, even in a population with a low prevalence of infection. If the Western blot test result is indeterminant, the testing sequence is considered equivocal for HIV infection. When this occurs, the Western blot test should be repeated on the same serum sample, and, if still indeterminant, the testing sequences should be repeated on a sample collected 3-6 months later. Use of other supplemental tests may aid in interpreting of results on samples that are persistently indeterminant by Western blot.

Testing of Patients

Previous CDC recommendations have emphasized the value of HIV serologic testing of patients for: (1) management of parenteral or mucous-membrane exposures of health-care workers, (2) patient diagnosis and management, and (3) counseling and serologic testing to prevent and control HIV transmission in the community. In addition, more recent recommendations have stated that hospitals, in conjunction with state and local health departments, should periodically determine the prevalence of HIV infection among patients from age groups at highest risk of infection (CDC, 1987).

Adherence to universal blood and body-fluid precautions recommended for the care of all patients will minimize the risk of transmission of HIV and other blood-borne pathogens from patients to health-care workers. The utility of routine HIV serologic testing of patients as an adjunct to universal precautions is unknown. Results of such testing may not be available in emergency or outpatient settings. In addition, some recently infected patients will not have detectable antibody to HIV.

Personnel in some hospitals have advocated serologic testing of patients in settings in which exposure of health-care workers to large amounts of patients' blood may be anticipated. Specific patients for whom serologic testing has been advocated include those undergoing major operative procedures and those undergoing treatment in critical-care units, especially if they have conditions involving uncontrolled bleeding. Decisions regarding the need to establish testing programs for patients should be made by physicians or individual institutions. In addition, when deemed appropriate, testing of individual patients may be performed on agreement between the patient and the physician providing care.

In addition to the universal precautions recommended for all patients, certain additional precautions for the care of HIV-infected patients undergoing major surgical operations have been proposed by personnel in some hospitals. For example, surgical procedures on an HIV-infected patient might be altered so that hand-to-hand passing of sharp instruments would be eliminated; stapling instruments rather than hand-suturing equipment might be used to perform tissue approximation; electrocautery devices rather than scalpels might be used as cutting instruments; and, even though uncomfortable, gowns that totally prevent seepage of blood onto the skin of members of the operative team might be worn. While such modifications might further minimize the risk of HIV infection for members of the operative team, some of these techniques could result in prolongation of operative time and could potentially have an adverse effect on the patient.

Testing programs, if developed, should include the following principles:

- Obtaining consent for testing
- Informing patients of test results, and providing counseling for seropositive patients by properly trained persons
- Assuring that confidentiality safeguards are in place to limit knowledge of test results to those directly involved in the care of infected patients or as required by law
- Assuring that identification of infected patients will not result in denial of needed care or provision of suboptimal care
- Evaluating prospectively 1) the efficacy of the program in reducing the incidence of parenteral, mucous-membrane, or significant cutaneous exposures of health-care workers to the blood or other body fluids of HIV-infected patients and 2) the effect of modified procedures on patients

TESTING OF HEALTH-CARE WORKERS

Although transmission of HIV from infected health-care workers to patients has not been reported, transmission during invasive procedures remains a possibility. Transmission of hepatitis B virus (HBV)— a blood-borne agent with a considerably greater potential for nosocomial spread—from health-care workers to patients has been documented. Such transmission has occurred in situations (e.g., oral and gynecologic surgery) in which health-care workers, when tested, had very high concentrations of HBV in their blood (at least 100 million infectious virus particles per milliliter, a concentration much higher than occurs with HIV infection), and the health-care workers sustained a puncture wound while performing invasive procedures or had exudative or weeping lesions or microlacerations that allowed virus to contaminate instruments or open wounds of patients (Kane & Lettau, 1985; Williams, 1983).

The hepatitis B experience indicates that only those health-care workers who perform certain types of invasive procedures have transmitted HBV to patients. Adherence to recommendations in this document will minimize the risk of transmission of HIV and other blood-borne pathogens from health-care workers to patients during invasive procedures. Since transmission of HIV from infected health-care workers performing invasive procedures to their patients has not been reported and would be expected to occur only very rarely, if at all, the utility of routine testing of such health-care workers to prevent transmission of HIV cannot be assessed. If consideration is given to developing a serologic testing program for health-care workers who perform invasive procedures, the frequency of testing, as well as the issues of consent, confidentiality, and consequences of test results—as previously outlined for testing programs for patients—must be addressed.

MANAGEMENT OF INFECTED HEALTH-CARE WORKERS

Health-care workers with impaired immune systems resulting from HIV infection or other causes are at increased risk of acquiring or experiencing serious complications of infectious disease. Of particular concern is the risk of severe infection following exposure to patients with infectious diseases that are easily transmitted if appropriate precautions are not taken (e.g., measles, varicella). Any health-care worker with an impaired immune system should be counseled about the potential risk associated with taking care of patients with any transmissible infection and should continue to follow existing recommendations for infection control to minimize risk of exposure to other infectious agents (Garner & Simmons, 1983: Williams, 1983). Recommendations of the Immunization Practices Advisory Committee (ACIP) and institutional policies concerning requirements for vaccinating health-care workers with live-virus vaccines (e.g., measles, rubella) should also be considered.

The question of whether workers infected with HIV—especially those who perform invasive procedures—can adequately and safely be allowed to perform patient-care duties or whether their work assignments should be changed must be determined on an individual basis. These decisions should be made by the health-care worker's personal physician(s) in conjunction with the medical director and personnel health service staff of the employing institution or hospital.

MANAGEMENT OF EXPOSURES

If a health-care worker has a parenteral (e.g., needlestick or cut) or mucous-membrane (e.g., splash to the eye or mouth) exposure to blood or other body fluids or has a cutaneous exposure involving large amounts of blood or prolonged contact with blood—especially when the exposed skin is chapped, abraded, or afflicted with dermatitis—the source patient should be informed of the incident and tested for serologic evidence of HIV infection after consent is obtained. Policies should be developed for testing source patients in situations in which consent cannot be obtained (e.g., an unconscious patient).

If the source patient has AIDS, is positive for HIV antibody, or refuses the test, the health-care workers should be counseled regarding the risk of infection and evaluated clinically and serologically for evidence of HIV infection as soon as possible after the exposure. The health-care worker should be advised to report and seek medical evaluation for any acute febrile illness that occurs within 12 weeks after the exposure. Such an illness—particularly one characterized by fever, rash, or lymphadenopathy—may be indicative of recent HIV infection. Seronegative health-care workers should be retested 6 weeks post-exposure and on a periodic basis thereafter (e.g., 12 weeks and 6 months after exposure) to determine whether transmission has occurred. During this follow-up period—especially the first 6–12 weeks after exposure, when most infected persons are expected to seroconvert—exposed health-care workers should follow U.S. Public Health Service (PHS) recommendations for preventing transmission of HIV (CDC, 1983b, 1985a).

No further follow-up of a health-care worker exposed to infection as described above is necessary if the source patient is seronegative unless the source patient is at high risk of HIV infection. In the latter case, a subsequent specimen (e.g., 12 weeks following exposure) may be obtained from the health-care worker for antibody testing. If the source patient cannot be identified, decisions regarding appropriate follow-up should be individualized. Serologic testing should be available to all health-care workers who are concerned that they may have been infected with HIV.

If a patient has a parenteral or mucous-membrane exposure to blood or other body fluid of a health-care worker, the patient should be informed of the incident, and the same procedure outlined above for management of exposures should be followed for both the source health-care worker and the exposed patient.

REFERENCES

Anonymous (1984) Needlestick transmission of HTLV-III from a patient infected in Africa. *Lancet* 2:1376–1377.

Baker, J. L, G. D. Kelen, K. T. Sivertson & T. C. Quinn, (1987) Unsuspected human immunodeficiency virus in critically ill emergency patients, *Journal of the American Medical Association* 257:2609–2611.

CDC (1982) Acquired immunodeficiency syndrome (AIDS): Precautions for clinical and laboratory staffs. *Morbidity and Mortality Weekly Report* 31:577–580.

CDC (1983a) Acquired immunodeficiency syndrome (AIDS). Precautions for health-care workers and allied professionals. *Morbidity and Mortality Weekly Report* 32:450–451.

CDC (1983b) Prevention of acquired immune deficiency syndrome (AIDS): Report of inter-agency recommendations. *Morbidity and Mortality Weekly Report* 32:101–103.

CDC (1985a) Provisional Public Health Service inter-agency recommendations for screening donated blood and plasma for antibody to the virus causing acquired immunodeficiency syndrome. *Morbidity and Mortality Weekly Report* 34:1–5.

CDC (1985b) Recommendations for preventing possible transmission of human T-lymphotropic virus type III/lymphadenopathy-associated virus from tears. *Morbidity and Mortality Weekly Report* 34:533–534.

CDC (1985c) Recommendations for preventing transmission of infection with human T-lymphotropic virus type III/lymphadenopathy-associated virus in the workplace. *Morbidity and Mortality Weekly Report* 34:681-686, 691–695.

CDC (1986a) Apparent transmission of human T-lymphotropic virus type III/lymphadenopathy-associated virus from a child to a mother providing health care. *Morbidity and Mortality Weekly Report* 35:76–79.

CDC (1986b) Human T-lymphotropic virus type III/lymphadenopathy-associated virus: Agent summary statement. *Morbidity and Mortality Weekly Report* 35:540-542, 547–549.

CEC (1986c) Recommendations for preventing transmission of infection with human T-lymphotropic virus type III/lymphadenopathy-associated virus during invasive procedures. *Morbidity and Mortality Weekly Report* 35:221–223.

CDC (1986d) Recommendations for providing dialysis treatment to patients infected with human T-lymphotropic virus type III/lymphadenopathy-associated virus infection. *Morbidity and Mortality Weekly Report* 35:376–378, 383.

CDC (1986e) Recommended infection control practices for dentistry. *Morbidity and Mortality Weekly Report* 35:237–242.

CDC (1987a) Public Health Service (PHS) guidelines for counseling and antibody testing to prevent HIV infection and AIDS. *Morbidity and Mortality Weekly Report* 3:509–515.

CDC (1987b) Update: Human immunodeficiency virus infections in health-care workers exposed to blood of infected patients. *Morbidity and Mortality Weekly Report* 36:285–289.

Environmental Protection Agency (1986) *EPA Guide for Infectious Waste Management* (Publication No. EPA/530-SW-86-014). Washington, DC: U. S. Environmental Protection Agency.

Favero, M. S. (1985) Sterilization, disinfection, and antisepsis in the hospital. In *Manual of Clinical Microbiology*, 4th ed., pp. 129–137. Washington, DC: American Society for Microbiology.

Favero, M. S. (1985) Dialysis-associated diseases and their control. In J. V. Bennett & P. S. Brachman, eds., *Hospital Infections*, pp. 267–84. Boston: Little, Brown and Company.

Garner, J. S. & M. S. Favero (1985) *Guideline for Handwashing and Hospital Environmental Control* (DHHS Publication No. 99–1117). Atlanta: Public Health Service, Centers for Disease Control.

Garner, J. S. & B. P. Simmons (1983) Guidelines for isolation precautions in hospitals. *Infection Control* 4(suppl.):245–325.

Gerberding, J. L., C. E. Bryant-LeBlanc, K. Nelson, et al. (1987) Risk of transmitting the human immunodeficiency virus, cytomegalovirus, and hepatitits B virus to health-care workers exposed to patients with AIDS and AIDS-related conditions. *Journal of Infectious Disease* 156:1–8.

Grint, P. & M. McEvoy (1985) Two associated cases of the acquired immune deficiency syndrome (AIDS). *PHLS Communicable Disease Report* 42:4.

Henderson, D. K., A. J. Saah, B. J. Zak, et al. (1986) Risk of nosocomial infection with human T-cell lymphotropic virus type III/lymphadenopathy-associated virus in a large cohort of intensively exposed health-care workers. *Annals of Internal Medicine* 104:644–647.

Kane, M. A. & L. A. Lettau (1985) Transmission of HBV from dental personnel to patients. *Journal of the American Medical Association* 255:934–937.

Kline, R. S., J. Phelan, G. H. Friedland, et al. (1985) Low occupational risk for HIV infection for dental professionals {Abstract}. In Abstracts from the Third International Conference on AIDS, 1985. Washington, D.C.

Martin, L. S., J. S. McDougal & S. L. Loskoski (1985) Disinfection and inactivation of the human T-lymphotropic virus type III/lymphadenopathy-associated virus. *Journal of Infectious Disease*, 152, 400–403.

McCray, E. (1986) The cooperative needlestick surveillance group. Occupational risk of the acquired immunodeficiency syndrome among health-care workers. *New England Journal of Medicine* 314:1127–1132.

McDougal, J., L. Martin, S. Cort., et al. (1985). Thermal inactivation of the acquired immunodeficiency syndrome virus-III/lymphadenopathy-associated virus, with special reference to antihemophiliac factor. *Journal of Clinical Investigation, 76,* 875–877.

McEvoy, M., K. Porter, P. Mortimer, N. Simmons & D. Shanson (1987) Prospective study of clinical, laboratory, and ancillary staff with accidental exposures to blood or other body fluids from patients infected with HIV. *British Medical Journal* 294:1595–1597.

Neisson-Vernant, C., S. Arfi, D. Mathez, J. Leibowitch & N. Monplaisir (1986) Needlestick HIV seroconversion in a nurse. *Lancet* 2:814.

Oksenhendler, E., M. Harzic, J. M. Le Roux, C. Rabian & J. P. Clauvel (1986) HIV infection with seroconversion after a superficial needlestick injury to the finger. *New England Journal of Medicine* 315:582.

Resnik, L., K. Veren, S. Z. Salahuddin, S. Tondreau & P. D. Markham (1986) Stability and inactivation of HTLV III/LAV under clinical and laboratory environments. *Journal of the American Medical Association* 255:1887–1891.

Richardson, J. H. & W. E. Barkley, eds. (1984) *Biosafety in microbiological and biomedical laboratories* (DHHS Publication No. [CDC] 84-8395). Washington, DC: U.S. Department of Health and Human Services, Public Health Service.

Spire, B., F. Barre-Sinoussi, D. Dormont, L. Montagnier & J. C. Chermann (1985) Inactivation of lymphadenopathy-associated virus by heat, gamma rays, and ultraviolet light. *Lancet* 1:188–189.

Spire, B., L. Montagnier, F. Barre-Sinoussi & J. C. Chermann (1984) Inactivation of lymphadenopathy-associated virus by chemical disinfectants. *Lancet* 2:899–901.

Williams, W. W. (1983) Guideline for infection control in hospital personnel. *Infection Control* 4(suppl.):326–349.

APPENDIX G

Update: Universal Precautions for Prevention of Transmission of Human Immunodeficiency Virus, Hepatitis B Virus, and Other Bloodborne Pathogens in Health-Care Settings

INTRODUCTION

The purpose of this report is to clarify and supplement the CDC publication entitled "Recommendations for Prevention of HIV Transmission in Health-Care Settings" (CDC, 1987).

In 1983, CDC published a document entitled "Guidelines for Isolation Precautions in Hospitals" that contained a section entitled "Blood and Body Fluid Precautions." The recommendations in this section called for blood and body fluid precautions when a patient was known or suspected to be infected with bloodborne pathogens (Garner & Simmons, 1983). In August 1987, CDC published a document entitled "Recommendations for Prevention of HIV Transmission in Health-Care Settings" (CDC, 1987). In contrast to the 1983 document, the 1987 document recommended that blood and body fluid precautions be consistently used for all patients regardless of their bloodborne infection status. This extension of blood and body fluid precautions to all patients is referred to as "Universal Blood and Body Fluid Precautions" or "Universal Precautions." Under universal precautions, blood and certain body fluids of all patients are considered potentially infectious for human immunodeficiency virus (HIV), hepatitis B virus (HBV), and other bloodborne pathogens.

Morbidity and Mortality Weekly Report 37(24), June 24, 1988, 377–388.

Universal precautions are intended to prevent parenteral, mucous-membrane, and nonintact skin exposures of health-care workers to bloodborne pathogens. In addition, immunization with HBV vaccine is recommended as an important adjunct to universal precautions for health-care workers who have exposures to blood (DOL/DHHS, 1987; Immunization Practices Advisory Group, 1985).

Since the recommendations for universal precautions were published in August 1987, CDC and the Food and Drug Administration (FDA) have received requests for clarification of the following issues: (1) body fluids to which universal precautions apply, (2) use of protective barriers, (3) use of gloves for phlebotomy, (4) selection of gloves for use while observing universal precautions, and (5) need for making changes in waste management programs as a result of adopting universal precautions.

BODY FLUIDS TO WHICH UNIVERSAL PRECAUTIONS APPLY

Universal precautions apply to blood and to other body fluids containing visible blood. Occupational transmission of HIV and HBV to health-care workers by blood is documented (CDC, 1988; DOL/DHHS, 1987). *Blood is the single most important source of HIV, HBV, and other bloodborne pathogens in the occupational setting.* Infection control efforts for HIV, HBV, and other bloodborne pathogens must focus on preventing exposures to blood as well as on delivery of HBV immunization.

Universal precautions also apply to semen and vaginal secretions. Although both of these fluids have been implicated in the sexual transmission of HIV and HBV, they have not been implicated in occupational transmission from patient to health-care worker. This observation is not unexpected, since exposure to semen in the usual health-care setting is limited, and the routine practice of wearing gloves for performing vaginal examinations protects health-care workers from exposure to potentially infectious vaginal secretions.

Universal precautions also apply to tissues and to the following fluids: cerebrospinal fluid (CSF), synovial fluid, pleural fluid, peritoneal fluid, pericardial fluid, and amniotic fluid. The risk of transmission of HIV and HBV from these fluids is unknown; epidemiologic studies in the health-care and community setting are currently inadequate to assess the potential risk to health-care workers from occupational exposures to them. However, HIV has been isolated from CSF, synovial, and amniotic fluid (Hollander & Levy, 1987; Mundy, Schinazi, Gerber, Nahmias & Randall, 1987; Wirthington, Cornes, Harris, et al., 1987), and HBsAg has been detected in synovial fluid, amniotic fluid, and peritoneal fluid (Bond, Petersen, Gravelle & Favero, 1982; Lee, Ip & Wong, 1978; Onion, Crumpacker & Gilliland, 1971). One case of HIV transmission was reported after a percutaneous exposure to bloody pleural fluid obtained by needle aspiration (Oskenhendler, Harzic, Le Roux, Rabian & Clauvel, 1986). Whereas aseptic procedures used to obtain these fluids for diagnostic or therapeutic purposes protect health-care workers from skin exposures, they cannot prevent penetrating injuries due to contaminated needles or other sharp instruments.

BODY FLUIDS TO WHICH UNIVERSAL PRECAUTIONS DO NOT APPLY

Universal precautions do not apply to feces, nasal secretions, sputum, sweat, tears, urine, and vomitus unless they contain visible blood. The risk of transmission of HIV and HBV from these fluids and materials is extremely low or nonexistent. HIV has been isolated and HBsAg has been demonstrated in some of these fluids; however, epidemiologic studies in the health-care and community settings have not implicated these fluids or materials in the transmission of HIV and HBV infections (Friedland, Saltzman, Rogers, et al., 1986; Lifson, 1988). Some of the above fluids and excretions represent a potential source for nosocomial and community-acquired infections with other pathogens, and recommendations for preventing the transmission of nonbloodborne pathogens have been published (Garner & Simmons, 1983).

PRECAUTIONS FOR OTHER BODY FLUIDS IN SPECIAL SETTINGS

Human breast milk has been implicated in perinatal transmission of HIV, and HBsAg has been found in the milk of mothers infected with HBV (Lee, Ip & Wong, 1978; Lifson, 1988). However, occupational exposure to human breast milk has not been implicated in the transmission of HIV nor HBV infection to health-care workers. Moreover, the health-care worker will not have the same type of intensive exposure to breast milk as the nursing neonate. Whereas universal precautions do not apply to human breast milk, gloves may be worn by health-care workers in situations where exposures to breast milk might be frequent, for example, in breast milk banking.

Saliva of some persons infected with HBV has been shown to contain HBV-DNA at concentrations 1/1,000 to 1/10,000 of that found in the infected person's serum (Jenison, Lemon, Baker & Newbold, 1987). HBsAg-positive saliva has been shown to be infectious when injected into experimental animals and in human bite exposures (Cancio-Bello, de Medina, Shorey, Valledor & Schiff, 1982; MacQuarrie, Forghani & Wolochow, 1974; Scott, Snitbhan, Bancroft, Alter & Tingpalapong, 1980). However, HBsAg-positive saliva has not been shown to be infectious when applied to oral mucous membranes in experimental primate studies or through contamination of musical instruments or cardiopulmonary resuscitation dummies used by HBV carriers (Scott, Snitbhan, Bancroft & Alter, 1980; Glaser & Nadler, 1985; Osterholm, Bravo, Crosson, et al., 1979). Epidemiologic studies of nonsexual household contacts of HIV-infected patients, including several small series in which HIV transmission failed to occur after bites or after percutaneous inoculation or contamination of cuts and open wounds with saliva from HIV-infected patients, suggest that the potential for salivary transmission of HIV is remote (CDC, 1988; Curran, Jaffe, Hardy, et al., 1988; Friedland, Saltzman, Rogers, et al., 1986; Jason, McDougal, Dixon, et al., 1986). One case report from Germany has suggested the possibility of transmission of HIV in a household setting from an infected child to a sibling through a human bite (Wahn, Kramer, Voit, Bruster, Scrampical & Scheid, 1986). The bite did not break the skin or result in bleeding. Since the date of seroconversion to HIV was not known for either child in this case, evidence for the role of saliva in the transmission of virus is unclear. Another case report suggested the possibility of transmission of HIV from husband to wife by contact with saliva during kissing (Salahuddin, Groopman, Markham, et al., 1984). However, follow-up studies did not confirm HIV infection in the wife (Curran, Jaffe, Hardy et al., 1988).

Universal precautions do not apply to saliva. General infection control practices already in existence — including the use of gloves for digital examination of mucous membranes and endotracheal suctioning, and handwashing after exposure to saliva — could further minimize the minute risk, if any, for salivary transmission of HIV and HBV (CDC, 1988; Klein, Phelan, Freeman, et al., 1988). During dental procedures, contamination of saliva with blood is predictable, trauma to health-care workers' hands is common, and blood spattering may occur. Infection control precautions for dentistry minimize the potential for nonintact skin and mucous membrane contact of dental health-care workers to blood-contaminated saliva of patients. In addition, the use of gloves for oral examinations and treatment in the dental setting may also protect the patient's oral mucous membranes from exposures to blood, which may occur from breaks in the skin of dental workers' hands.

USE OF PROTECTIVE BARRIERS

Protective barriers reduce the risk of exposure of the health-care worker's skin or mucous membranes to potentially infective materials. For universal precautions, protective barriers reduce the risk of exposure to blood, body fluids containing visible blood, and other fluids to which universal precautions apply. Examples of protective barriers include gloves, gowns, masks, and protective eyewear. Gloves should reduce the incidence of contamination of hands, but they cannot prevent penetrating injuries due to needles or other sharp instruments. Masks and protective eyewear or face shields should reduce the incidence of contamination of mucous membranes of the mouth, nose, and eyes.

Universal precautions are intended to supplement rather than replace recommendations for routine infection control, such as handwashing and using gloves to prevent gross microbial contamination of hands (Garner & Favero, 1985). Because specifying the types of barriers needed for every possible clinical situation is impractical, some judgment must be exercised.

The risk of nosocomial transmission of HIV, HBV, and other blood-borne pathogens can be minimized if health-care workers use the following general guidelines:

1. Take care to prevent injuries when using needles, scalpels, and other sharp instruments or devices; when handling sharp instruments after procedures; when cleaning used instruments; and when disposing of used needles. Do not recap used needles by

hand; do not remove used needles from disposable syringes by hand; and do not bend, break, or otherwise manipulate used needles by hand. Place used disposable syringes and needles, scalpel blades, and other sharp items in puncture-resistant containers for disposal. Locate the puncture-resistant containers as close to the use area as is practical.

2. Use protective barriers to prevent exposure to blood, body fluids containing visible blood, and other fluids to which universal precautions apply. The type of protective barrier(s) should be appropriate for the procedure being performed and the type of exposure anticipated.

3. Immediately and thoroughly wash hands and other skin surfaces that are contaminated with blood, body fluids containing visible blood, or other body fluids to which universal precautions apply.

GLOVE USE FOR PHLEBOTOMY

Gloves should reduce the incidence of blood contamination of hands during phlebotomy (drawing blood samples), but they cannot prevent penetrating injuries caused by needles or other sharp instruments. The likelihood of hand contamination with blood containing HIV, HBV, or other bloodborne pathogens during phlebotomy depends on several factors: 1) the skill and technique of the health-care workers, 2) the frequency with which the health-care worker performs the procedure (other factors being equal, the cumulative risk of blood exposure is higher for a health-care worker who performs more procedures), 3) whether the procedure occurs in a routine or emergency situation (where blood contact may be more likely), and 4) the prevalence of infection with bloodborne pathogens in the patient population. The likelihood of infection after skin exposure to blood containing HIV or HBV will depend on the concentration of virus (viral concentration is much higher for hepatitis B than for HIV), the duration of contact, the presence of skin lesions on the hands of the health-care worker, and —for HBV—the immune status of the health-care worker. Although not accurately quantified, the risk of HIV infection following intact skin contact with infective blood is certainly much less than the 0.5% risk following percutaneous needlestick exposures (CDC, 1988). In universal precautions, all blood is assumed to be potentially infective for bloodborne pathogens, but in certain settings (e.g., volunteer blood-donation centers) the prevalence of infection with some bloodborne pathogens (e.g., HIV, HBV) is known to be very low. Some institutions have relaxed recommendations for using gloves for phlebotomy procedures by skilled phlebotomists in settings where the prevalence of bloodborne pathogens is known to be very low.

Institutions that judge that routine gloving for all phlebotomies is not necessary should periodically reevaluate their policy. Gloves should always be available to health-care workers who wish to use them for phlebotomy. In addition, the following general guidelines apply:

1. Use gloves for performing phlebotomy when the health-care worker has cuts, scratches, or other breaks in his/her skin.
2. Use gloves in situations where the health-care worker judges that hand contamination with blood may occur, for example, when performing phlebotomy on an uncooperative patient.
3. Use gloves for performing finger and/or heel sticks on infants and children.
4. Use gloves when persons are receiving training in phlebotomy.

SELECTION OF GLOVES

The Center for Devices and Radiological Health, FDA, has responsibility for regulating the medical glove industry. Medical gloves include those marketed as sterile surgical or non-sterile examination gloves made of vinyl or latex. General purpose utility ("rubber") gloves are also used in the health-care setting, but they are not regulated by FDA since they are not promoted for medical use. There are no reported differences in barrier effectiveness between intact latex and intact vinyl used to manufacture gloves. Thus, the type of gloves selected should be appropriate for the task being performed.

The following general guidelines are recommended:

1. Use sterile gloves for procedures involving contact with normally sterile areas of the body.
2. Use examination gloves for procedures involving contact with mucous membranes, unless otherwise indicated, and for other patient care or diagnostic procedures that do not require the use of sterile gloves.
3. Change gloves between patient contacts.

4. Do not wash or disinfect surgical or examination gloves for reuse. Washing with surfactants may cause "wicking," i.e., the enhanced penetration of liquids through undetected holes in the glove. Disinfecting agents may cause deterioration.

5. Use general-purpose utility gloves (e.g., rubber household gloves) for housekeeping chores involving potential blood contact and for instrument cleaning and decontamination procedures. Utility gloves may be decontaminated and reused but should be discarded if they are peeling, cracked, or discolored, or if they have punctures, tears, or other evidence of deterioration.

WASTE MANAGEMENT

Universal precautions are not intended to change waste management programs previously recommended by CDC (1987) for health-care settings. Policies for defining, collecting, storing, decontaminating, and disposing of infective waste are generally determined by institutions in accordance with state and local regulations. Information regarding waste management regulations in health-care settings may be obtained from state or local health departments or agencies responsible for waste management.

Editorial Note: Implementation of universal precautions does not eliminate the need for other category- or disease-specific isolation precautions, such as enteric precautions for infectious diarrhea or isolation for pulmonary tuberculosis (CDC, 1987; Garner & Simmons, 1983). In addition to universal precautions, detailed precautions have been developed for the following procedures and/or settings in which prolonged or intensive exposures to blood occur: invasive procedures, dentistry, autopsies or morticians' services, dialysis, and the clinical laboratory. These detailed precautions are found in the August 21, 1987, "Recommendations for Prevention of HIV Transmission in Health-Care Settings" (CDC, 1987). In addition, specific precautions have been developed for research laboratories (CDC, 1988).

REFERENCES

Bond, W. W., N. J. Petersen, C. R. Gravelle & M. S. Favero (1982) Hepatitis B virus in peritoneal dialysis fluid: A potential hazard. *Dialysis and Transplantation* 11:592–600.

Cancio-Bello, T. P., M. de Medina, J. Shorey, M. D. Valledor & E. R. Schiff (1982) An institutional outbreak of hepatitis B related to a human biting carrier. *Journal of Infectious Disease* 146:652–656.

Centers for Disease Control (1987) Recommendations for prevention of HIV transmission in health-care settings. *Morbidity and Mortality Weekly Report* 36(suppl. no. 2S).

Centers for Disease Control (1988) Update: Acquired immunodeficiency syndrome and human immunodeficiency virus infection among health-care workers. *Morbidity and Mortality Weekly Report* 294:484.

Curran, J. W., H. W. Jaffe, A. M. Hardy, et al. (1988) Epidemiology of HIV infection and AIDS in the United States. *Science* 239:610–616.

Department of Labor, Department of Health and Human Services. (1987) Joint advisory notice; protection against occupational exposure to hepatitis B virus (HBV) and human immunodeficiency virus (HIV). Washington, DC: U.S. Department of Labor, U.S. Department of Health and Human Services.

Friedland, G. H., B. R. Saltzman, M. F. Rogers, et al. (1986) Lack of transmission of HTLV-III/LAV infection to household contacts of patients with AIDS or AIDS-related complex with oral candidiasis. *New England Journal of Medicine* 314:344–349.

Garner, J. S., & M.S. Favero, (1985). Guideline for Handwashing and hospital environmental control. Atlanta: DHHS, PHS, CDC. Publication No. 99–117.

Garner, J. S., & B. P. Simmons (1983) Guideline for isolation precautions in hospitals. *Infection control* 4:245–325.

Glaser, J. B., & J. P. Nadler (1985) Hepatitis B virus in a cardiopulmonary resuscitation training course: Risk of transmission from a surface antigen-positive participant. *Archives of Internal Medicine* 145:1653–1655.

Hollander, H., & J. A. Levy (1987) Neurologic abnormalities and recovery of human immunodeficiency virus from synovial fluid of a patient with reactive arthritis. *British Medical Journal* 294:484.

Immunization Practices Advisory Committee (1985) Recommendations for protection against viral hepatitis. *Morbidity and Mortality Weekly Report* 34:313–324, 329–335.

Jason, J. M., J. S. McDougal, G. Dixon, et al. (1986) HTLV-III/LAV antibody and immune status of household contacts and sexual partners of persons with hemophilia. *Journal of the American Medical Association* 255:212–215.

Jenison, S. A., S. M. Lemon, L. N. Baker & J. E. Newbold (1987) Quantitative analysis of hepatitis B virus DNA in saliva and semen of chronically infected homosexual men. *Journal of Infectious Disease* 156:299–306.

Klein, R.S., J.A. Phelan, K. Freeman, et al. (1985). Low occupational risk of human immunodeficiency virus infection among dental professionals. *New England Journal of Medicine*, 318, 86–90.

Lee, A. K. Y., H. M. H. Ip & V. C. W. Wong (1978) Mechanisms of maternal-fetal transmission of hepatitis B virus. *Journal of Infectious Disease* 138:668–671.

Lifson, A. R. (1988) Do alternate modes for transmission of human immunodeficiency virus exist? A review. *Journal of the American Medical Association* 259:1353–1356.

MacQuarrie, M. B., B. Forghani, D & A. Wolochow (1974) Hepatitis B transmitted by a human bite. *Journal of the American Medical Association* 230:723–724.

Mundy, D. C., R. F. Schinazi, A. R. Gerber, A.J. Nahmias & H. W. Randall (1987) Human immunodeficiency virus isolated from amniotic fluid. *Lancet* 2:459–460.

Onion, D. D., C. S. Crumpacker & B. C. Gilliland (1971) Arthritis of hepatitis associated with Australia antigen. *Annals of Internal Medicine* 75:29–33.

Oskenhendler, E., M. Harzic, J. M. Le Roux, C. Rabian & J. P. Clauvel (1986) HIV infection with seroconversion after a superficial needlestick injury to the finger [Letter]. *New England Journal of Medicine* 315:582.

Osterholm, M. T., E. R. Bravo, J. T. Crosson, et al. (1979) Lack of transmission of viral hepatitis type B after oral exposure to HBsAg-positive saliva. *British Medical Journal* 2:1263–1264.

Salahuddin, S. Z., J. E. Groopman, P. D. Markham, et al. (1984) HTLV-III in symptom-free seronegative persons. *Lancet* 2:1418–1420.

Scott, R. M., R. Snitbhan, W. H. Bancroft, H. J. Alter & M. Tingpalapong (1980) Experimental transmission of hepatitis B virus by semen and saliva. *Journal of Infectious Disease* 146:652–656.

Simmons, B. P., & E. S. Wong (1982) *Guidelines for Prevention of Nosocomial Pneumonia.* Atlanta: U.S. Department of Health and Human Services, Public Health Service, Centers for Disease Control.

Wahn, V., H. H. Kramer, T. Voit, H. T. Bruster, B. Scrampical & A. Scheid (1986) Horizontal transmission of HIV infection between two siblings [Letter]. *Lancet* 2:694.

Wirthington, R. H., P. Cornes, J.R. Harris, et al. (1987). Isolation of human immunodeficiency virus from synovial fluid of a patient with reactive arthritis. *British Medical Journal,* 294, 484.

APPENDIX H

Update: Acquired Immunodeficiency Syndrome (AIDS)—Worldwide

As of March 21, 1988, 136 countries or territories throughout the world had reported a total of 84,256 cases of acquired immunodeficiency syndrome (AIDS) to the Gloval Programme on AIDS (GPA)(formerly the Special Programme on AIDS) of the World Health Organization (WHO)(Table H-1). Because of varying reporting practices, AIDS case data are not available for all countries for the same time period. Thirty-seven countries or territories had reported no AIDS cases. Reports are based on either the CDC/WHO surveillance definition, the WHO clinical definition, or a physician's diagnosis (CDC, 1987; WHO, 1986, 1988). From 1979 through March 21, 1988, the number of AIDS cases increased markedly in all geographic regions. The cumulative world total increased from 11,965 in 1984 to 25,150 in 1985 (a 110% increase) and to 48,413 in 1986 (a 92% increase). Because of reporting lags, the global total of AIDS cases reported for 1987 is not yet complete; however, as of March 21, 1988, 34,913 cases had been reported for 1987 (a 72% increase). Data on the distribution of AIDS cases by region are presented below, followed by a discussion of the findings.

AMERICAS

Forty-two countries in the Americas have reported 73% of the world total of AIDS cases. As of March 21, 1988, the United States had reported a total of 54,233 cases. The case count in Brazil was

Morbidity and Mortality Weekly Report 37(18), May 13, 1988, 286-288, 293-295.

TABLE H-1 **AIDS CASES REPORTED TO THE WORLD HEALTH ORGANIZATION, BY CONTINENT, 1979–MARCH 21, 1988**

Continent	Number of Cases	Total Number of Countries Responding
Africa	10,973	50
Americas	61,602	44
Asia	231	37
Europe	10,616	28
Oceania	834	14

2,325; the number had increased from 801 at the end of June 1986 to 1,695 at the end of June 1987. Canada has reported a total of 1,517 cases. The following additional countries reported over 100 cases: Haiti (912), Mexico (713), Dominican Republic (352), Trinidad and Tobago (206), Bahamas (163), Colombia (153), Argentina (120), and Venezuela (101).

EUROPE

Twenty-eight countries in Europe have reported 13% of the world's total AIDS cases. Between December 1986 and December 1987, the number of cases reported from Europe to the WHO Collaborating Centre on AIDS in Paris, France, increased by 124% (Institut de Medicine, 1987). The greatest number of cases has been reported from France (3,073), the Federal Republic of Germany (1,669), Italy (1,411), the United Kingdom (1,227), and Spain (789). The highest rates per population size are in France, Switzerland, and Denmark. Four countries with over 100 cases (Austria, France, Italy, and Spain) reported increases of more than 100% between December 1986 and December 1987. The lowest rates were reported from the Eastern European countries.

Ninety-two percent of patients reported from Europe were European, 4% were African; 1% were from the Caribbean; and 3% were from other countries. The relative percentage of patients who have been reported from Europe but whose country of origin is Africa has been decreasing over the past 2 years.

The age distribution of patients in Europe (Table H-2) is similar to that in the United States except that Europe has a higher percentage of patients under 19 years of age (3% compared with 2%). Europe has a lower percentage of adult patients in the homosexual and homosexual/intravenous-drug-user transmission categories than the United States and a higher percentage in the heterosexual, blood-related, and undetermined/other categories (Table H-3). In addition, Europe has a higher percentage of pediatric patients in the hemophilia/coagulation-disorder category than the United States and a lower percentage with a parent with AIDS or at increased risk for AIDS.

Intravenous (IV) drug users account for 64% of adult patients in Italy and 53% of adult patients in Spain. Both countries together reported 66% of the IV-drug-related cases in Europe. In the following six countries reporting more than 50 cases, 75% or more of the patients were homosexual males: the Netherlands (88%), the United Kingdom (87%), Denmark (86%), Sweden (81%), Norway (79%), and the Federal Republic of Germany (76%).

AFRICA

Thirty-eight countries in the African Region have reported 13% of the world's total AIDS cases. Fifteen African countries reported more than 50 cases each. Zimbabwe and Zaire have each reported 300 to 500 cases, and Uganda, Tanzania, Congo, Kenya, Burundi, Rwanda, Malawi, and Zambia have each reported more than 500 cases. Central, eastern, and southern Africa have reported the largest number of cases. Although cases were first officially reported from Africa in the second half of 1982, over 70% of all cases (7,906) were reported in 1987.

OTHER AREAS

Oceania has reported a total of 834 AIDS cases; Asia, a total of 231 cases; and the eastern Mediterranean countries, 100 cases. The major reporting countries (greater than 20 cases) from these areas were

TABLE H-2 **AIDS CASES, BY AGE GROUP AND SEX—28 COUN-TRIES IN THE WORLD HEALTH ORGANIZATION'S EUROPEAN REGION, DECEMBER 31, 1987**

Age Group	Male	Female	Total	(%)
0-11 mos	40	48	88	(0.9)
1-4 yrs	52	48	100	(1.0)
5-9 yrs	24	7	31	(0.3)
10-14 yrs	29	3	32	(0.3)
15-19 yrs	77	14	91	(0.9)
20-29 yrs	2,325	551	2,876	(28.2)
30-39 yrs	3,440	255	3,695	(36.3)
40-49 yrs	2,031	72	2,103	(20.7)
50-59 yrs	736	53	789	(7.7)
> 60 yrs	281	52	333	(3.3)
Unknown	38	2	43 *	(0.4)
Total	9,073	1,105	10,181	(100.0)

*Sex of three patients is unknown.

Australia (758 cases), New Zealand (74), Japan (59), Qatar (32), and Turkey (21).

DISCUSSION

Worldwide AIDS surveillance is coordinated by GPA at WHO in Geneva. Reports are received from collaborating centers, including CDC in the United States, the WHO Collaborating Centre in Paris, and WHO regional offices and ministries of health. Accuracy and completeness of AIDS reporting vary in different areas of the world. In 1985, a review of death certificates in the United States suggested that 89% of AIDS cases meeting the surveillance definition were reported. In Africa, reporting has only recently started in some countries and is, therefore, incomplete. Consequently, the proportion of AIDS cases that are reported in Africa is unknown. The WHO clinical case definition, used in areas where the prevalence of HIV is high, has a specificity of over 90% (Colebunders, Mann, Francis et al., 1987).

Epidemiologic studies indicate three broad yet distinct geographic patterns of transmission. Pattern I is typical of industrialized countries with large numbers of reported AIDS cases, such as North America, Western Europe, Australia, New Zealand, and parts of Latin America. In these areas, most cases occur among homosexual or bisexual males and urban IV drug users. Heterosexual transmission is responsible for only a small percentage of cases but is increasing. Transmission due to exposure to blood and blood products occurred between the late 1970's and 1985 in these countries but has now been largely controlled through the self-deferral of persons at increased risk for AIDS and by routine blood screening for human immunodeficiency virus (HIV) antibody. The ratio of male to female patients ranges from 10:1 to 15:1, and, to date, perinatal transmission is relatively uncommon. Overall population seroprevalence is estimated to be less than 1% but has been measured at up to 50% in some groups practicing high-risk behaviors, such as IV drug users and men with multiple male sex partners.

Pattern II is observed in areas of central, eastern, and southern Africa and in some Caribbean countries. In these areas, most cases occur among heterosexuals; the male-to-female ratio is approximately 1:1; and perinatal transmission is relatively more common than in other areas. IV drug use and homosexual transmission either do not

TABLE H-3. **REPORTED AIDS CASES AMONG ADULT AND PEDIATRIC PATIENTS, BY TRANSMISSION CATEGORY—EUROPE, DECEMBER 31, 1987, AND UNITED STATES, JANUARY 4, 1988.***

Transmission Categories	Europe		United States	
Adult Patients	*No.*	*(%)*	*No.*	*(%)*
Homosexual/Bisexual Male	5,865	(59)	32,138	(65)
Intravenous Drug Use	1,944	(20)	8,511	(17)
Homosexual Male and IV Drug Use	259	(3)	3,726	(8)
Hemophilia/Coagulation Disorder	349	(4)	494	(1)
Heterosexual Contact	609	(6)	1,987	(4)
Transfusion	359	(4)	1,144	(2)
Other/Undetermined	545	(5)	1,515	(3)
Total	9,930	(100)	49,515	(100)
Adult Patients	*No.*	*(%)*	*No.*	*(%)*
Hemophilia/Coagulation Disorder	38	(15)	40	(5)
Parent with/at Risk for AIDS	170	(68)	577	(77)
Transfusion	38	(15)	99	(13)
Other/Undetermined	5	(2)	34	(5)
Total	251	(100)	750	(100)

*The latest data analysis available for Europe is for December 31, 1987. The January 4, 1988, U.S. analysis is used here because it most closely approximates the time frame of the European analysis.

occur or occur at a very low level. In a number of these countries, overall population seroprevalence is estimated at more than 1%, and, in a few urban areas, up to 25% of the sexually active age group is infected. Transmission through contaminated blood and blood products has been a significant problem and continues in those countries that have not yet implemented nationwide donor screening.

Pattern III is found in areas of Eastern Europe, the Middle East, Asia, and most of the Pacific. HIV appears to have been introduced into these areas in the early to mid-1980's, and only small numbers of cases have been reported. Homosexual and heterosexual transmission have only recently been documented. Generally, cases have occurred among persons who have traveled to endemic areas or who have had sexual contact with individuals from endemic areas, such as homosexual men and female prostitutes. A small number of cases due to receipt of imported blood products has been reported.

Under its charter, the World Health Assembly of WHO has authorized GPA to develop and coordinate a global strategy for AIDS prevention and control. As of March 1988, 115 member states had agreed to collaborate in supporting and developing short-term (less than 1 year) plans for AIDS control. Between February 1987 and March 1988, GPA provided over 250 consultant visits to assist countries in developing these plans.

WHO is conducting worldwide surveillance of AIDS, developing standardized methods for HIV serosurveys, and creating a Global Commission on AIDS to provide GPA with scientific and technical guidance. In addition, experts have met in Geneva to discuss a variety of HIV-related issues. Health promotion and HIV prevention strategies have also been developed. GPA is organizing a network of specimen banks for geographically and temporally representative retroviral isolates and sera. GPA is also collaborating with a working group of leading AIDS virologists to standardize the characterization of HIV and related human retroviruses.

Although the number of AIDS cases is expected to increase significantly over the next few years, there is growing confidence that the spread of HIV can be stopped. Stopping HIV infection, however, will require a commitment that goes beyond geographic boundaries. Education and the means to eliminate or modify risk factors and risk behaviors will be the key. The global control of AIDS will require both committed national AIDS programs and strong international coordination, cooperation, and leadership.

REFERENCES

Centers for Disease Control (1987) Revision of the CDC surveillance case definition for acquired immunodeficiency syndrome. *Morbidity and Mortality Weekly Report* 36(suppl 1S).
Colebunders, R., J. M. Mann, H. Francis, et al. (1987) Evaluation of a clinical case-definition of acquired immunodeficiency syndrome in Africa. *Lancet* 1:492–494.
Hardy, A. M., E. T. Starcher, W. M. Morgan, et al. (1987) Review of death certificates to assess completeness of AIDS case reporting. *Public Health Reports* 102:386–391.
Institut de Medicine et d'Epidemiologie Africaines et Tropicales. (1987) *AIDS Surveillance in Europe.* Paris: Institut de Medicine et d'Epidemiologie Africaines et Tropicales (Quarterly Report no. 16).
World Health Organization (1986) Acquired immunodeficiency syndrome (AIDS): WHO/CDC case definition for AIDS. *Weekly Epidemiologic Record* 61:69–73.
World Health Organization (1988) Acquired immunodeficiency syndrome (AIDS); WHO/CDC case definition for AIDS. *Weekly Epidemiologic Record* 63:1–7.

GLOSSARY

AIDS — The end stage manifestation of infection with human immunodeficiency virus, which destroys important components of the human immune system.

AIDS-RELATED DISEASES — A variety of chronic symptoms that occur in HIV-infected persons, but whose conditions may not meet the Centers for Disease Control's case definition of AIDS.

ANTIBODY — A unique protein produced by blood plasma cells to counteract or kill some specific infectious agent like a virus or bacteria.

ANTI-VIRAL — A substance such as AZT that acts to inhibit some aspect of a virus's life cycle.

AZT (AZIDOTHYMIDINE) — An antiviral drug currently used in some HIV-infected people to reduce the frequency and severity of infections.

CASUAL CONTACT — Day-to-day contact between HIV-infected persons and others at home, at work, or at school. This type of contact does not include sexual or needle-sharing interaction and therefore does not result in spread of HIV infection.

ELISA — The "enzyme-linked immunosorbent assay," a rapid screening test used to detect antibody to HIV.

EPIDEMIC — The occurrence of any given illness in an area that is in excess of normal expectation.

FALSE NEGATIVE — A negative test result for a condition that is actually present.

FALSE POSITIVE — A positive test result for a condition that is actually not present.

HEPATITIS-B — An inflammation of the liver caused by a virus that is spread by needle-sharing and sexual contact.

HUMAN IMMUNODEFICIENCY VIRUS (HIV) — A retrovirus believed to be the causative agent for AIDS and AIDS-related disorders in this country.

IMMUNOSUPPRESSED — A state of the body when the immune defenses do not work normally, usually as a result of illness or the administration of certain drugs used to fight cancer or prepare the body to accept transplanted donor organs.

INCUBATION PERIOD — The time interval between infection and appearance of the first symptoms.

INFECTION — A condition in which the body or some part of it is invaded by a disease-causing microorganism or virus that, under favorable conditions, multiplies and produces effects that are harmful. Localized infections (as opposed to systemic or bodywide) are usually accompanied by inflammation, but inflammation may occur without infection.

LYMPH NODES — Distributed throughout the body, and function as a type of filter for foreign material.

LYMPHADENOPATHY — An abnormal condition in which lymph nodes enlarge.

MICROORGANISMS (MICROBES) — A tiny living body not perceptible to the naked eye.

OPPORTUNISTIC INFECTIONS — Infections with any organism or microbe, but especially fungi and bacteria, that occur due to an altered immune system. These organisms do not usually cause disease in a person with a healthy immune system.

RETROVIRUS — Known to cause cancerlike illnesses in animals. A class of virus having the ability to transform their own genetic material, RNA, into DNA and thus incorporate themselves into the genetic structure of an infected cell.

SEROCONVERSION — The point at which antibodies to specific antigens are produced by B lymphocytes (a specialized blood cell) and become detectable in the blood.

SERONEGATIVE — Producing a negative reaction to a blood test.

SEROPOSITIVE — Producing a positive reaction to a blood test; for example, testing positive for the HIV-antibody test.

VIRUS — the smallest class of microbes, not visible without electron microscopy, and a parasite dependent on nutrients from host cells. They consist of a strand of either DNA or RNA but not both, separated by a protein covering.

WESTERN BLOT — More difficult to perform and more expensive than the ELISA, this is a test that involves the identification of antibodies against specific protein molecules.

INDEX